HOLISTIC NURSING CARE

Nurturing Mind, Body, and Spirit

Clara Henderson

Table of Contents

Chapter 3: Holistic Nursing Interventions

Chapter 4: Nurturing Emotional and Mental Health

Chapter 5: Fostering Spiritual and Existential Health

Chapter 6: Holistic Nursing in Special Populations

Chapter 7: Cultural Competence and Diversity in Holistic Care

Chapter 8: Holistic Self-Care for Nurses

Chapter 9:   Ethical Considerations in Holistic Nursing

Chapter 10: Holistic Nursing in the Future

Conclusion

Chapter 1:
Introduction to Holistic Nursing Care

Defining Holistic Nursing

Holistic nursing is a patient-centered approach to healthcare that emphasizes the integration of mind, body, and spirit in the delivery of care. It recognizes that individuals are complex beings with physical, emotional, mental, and spiritual dimensions, and it seeks to address the whole person rather than just their symptoms or illness. Holistic nurses consider not only the physical health of their patients but also their emotional well-being, mental health, and spiritual needs, striving to promote balance and harmony in all aspects of the patient's life. This approach involves therapeutic techniques and interventions that encompass a wide range of healing modalities, including conventional medicine, complementary therapies, and mind-body practices, with the ultimate goal of enhancing overall health and well-being.

Defining holistic nursing requires a comprehensive understanding of its principles, practices, and underlying philosophy. Detailed explanation of defining holistic nursing is given below:

Patient-Centered Approach: At the core of holistic nursing is a patient-centered approach. This means that the patient is viewed as a whole person rather than a collection of symptoms or diseases. Holistic nurses prioritize understanding the patient's unique needs, values, beliefs, and preferences.

Integration of Mind, Body, and Spirit: Holistic nursing recognizes that individuals are not just physical bodies but also have mental, emotional, and spiritual aspects. It emphasizes the integration of these dimensions in the delivery of care. This involves addressing emotional and psychological well-being, spiritual and existential concerns, and physical health simultaneously.

Assessment of All Dimensions: Holistic nurses conduct comprehensive assessments that encompass all dimensions of a patient's life. They not only assess physical symptoms but also inquire about emotional states, mental health, and spiritual or existential needs. This holistic assessment helps in creating a personalized care plan.

Emphasis on Prevention: Holistic nursing places a strong emphasis on preventive care. Nurses work with patients to identify risk factors, lifestyle choices, and stressors that may impact their health negatively. They promote strategies for maintaining and improving overall wellness.

Complementary Therapies: Holistic nursing incorporates complementary and alternative therapies into care when appropriate. These may include practices like acupuncture, massage therapy, yoga, meditation, and herbal medicine. The choice of therapies is based on the patient's preferences and needs.

Mind-Body Connection: Holistic nursing recognizes the interconnectedness of the mind and body. It understands that emotional and mental well-being can significantly impact physical health and vice versa. Nurses employ interventions that address this mind-body connection to promote healing.

Cultural Competence: Cultural sensitivity is a fundamental aspect of holistic nursing. Nurses respect and honor the cultural beliefs, values, and traditions of their patients, recognizing that these factors influence health and healing.

Patient Empowerment: Holistic nursing empowers patients to take an active role in their own care. Nurses collaborate with patients to set goals, make informed decisions, and participate in their healing process.

Communication and Therapeutic Relationships: Effective communication and the development of therapeutic relationships are key in holistic nursing. Nurses engage in active listening, empathy, and compassionate care to foster trust and collaboration with patients.

Spiritual and Existential Support: Holistic nurses provide support to patients in addressing spiritual and existential concerns. This may involve helping patients find meaning in their experiences, exploring their beliefs, or connecting with spiritual resources that offer comfort and strength.

Patient Education: Nurses educate patients about the various aspects of their care, including lifestyle choices, self-care practices, and the use of complementary therapies. Education empowers patients to make informed decisions about their health.

Wellness Promotion: Holistic nursing places a strong emphasis on promoting wellness rather than simply managing illness. Nurses work with patients to develop strategies for maintaining and enhancing their overall well-being.

Holistic nursing is a patient-centered and comprehensive approach to healthcare that recognizes the interconnectedness of mind, body, and spirit. It focuses on assessing and addressing all dimensions of a patient's life, emphasizing prevention, incorporating complementary therapies, and empowering patients to actively participate in their care. Holistic nurses aim to promote not only physical health but also emotional, mental, and spiritual well-being, ultimately facilitating holistic healing and wellness.

Historical Overview of Holistic Nursing

The historical development of holistic nursing traces the evolution of nursing from a primarily task-oriented profession to one that recognizes the importance of treating patients as whole beings with physical, emotional, mental, and spiritual dimensions. Here's a historical overview of holistic nursing:

Early Influences (19th Century): Nursing in the 19th century was primarily task-focused, emphasizing cleanliness, infection control, and basic patient care. However, notable pioneers like Florence Nightingale recognized the importance of the environment, nutrition, and emotional support in patient healing. Nightingale's emphasis on the psychological aspects of care laid the foundation for holistic nursing.

Holistic Health Movement (1950s-1960s): The holistic health movement in the mid-20th century played a significant role in shaping holistic nursing. Influential figures like Rachel Carson and Dr. Herbert Benson introduced concepts of mind-body-spirit interconnectedness and the impact of stress on health. This era marked the beginning of a more holistic approach to healthcare.

Founding of the American Holistic Nurses Association (AHNA) (1981): The establishment of the American Holistic Nurses Association was a pivotal moment in the development of holistic nursing. The AHNA promoted holistic principles, provided education and resources, and facilitated the incorporation of holistic care into nursing practice.

Nursing Theories and Models (1980s-1990s): Nurse theorists, such as Jean Watson and Martha Rogers, developed nursing models that emphasized holistic care, humanistic values, and the importance of the nurse-patient relationship. These theories contributed to the mainstream acceptance of holistic nursing concepts.

Holistic Nursing Certification (1986): The American Holistic Nurses Credentialing Corporation (AHNCC) was founded to establish certification standards for holistic nursing. This credentialing process helped legitimize holistic nursing as a specialized practice area.

Integration into Nursing Education (Late 20th Century - Present): Many nursing schools started to integrate holistic nursing principles into their curricula. This included education on complementary and alternative therapies, holistic assessment, and the importance of addressing emotional and spiritual aspects of care.

Research and Evidence-Based Practice: Holistic nursing has become a subject of research, with studies focusing on the impact of holistic interventions on patient outcomes.

This research has contributed to evidence-based practice guidelines that support holistic care approaches.

Modern Holistic Nursing (21st Century): In the 21st century, holistic nursing has continued to evolve. It embraces a wide range of practices, from incorporating complementary therapies like acupuncture and aromatherapy to promoting mindfulness and stress reduction techniques. Holistic nursing recognizes the value of cultural competence, diversity, and patient-centered care.

Integration into Mainstream Healthcare: Holistic nursing principles have been increasingly integrated into mainstream healthcare settings, including hospitals and clinics. This integration acknowledges the benefits of addressing patients' emotional, mental, and spiritual well-being alongside their physical health.

Continued Growth: Holistic nursing continues to grow as a field, with nurses specializing in areas like holistic nurse coaching, integrative healthcare, and wellness promotion. It remains responsive to the changing healthcare landscape and the evolving needs of patients.

The historical overview of holistic nursing reflects a journey from a task-oriented approach to a comprehensive, patient-centered model that recognizes the interconnectedness of mind, body, and spirit. It has been shaped by pioneers, nursing theories, certification standards, and ongoing research, making it an integral part of modern nursing practice. Holistic nursing not only addresses physical health but also places a strong emphasis on nurturing patients' emotional, mental, and spiritual well-being.

The Holistic Nursing Model

The Holistic Nursing Model is a framework that guides nurses in providing patient-centered care that takes into consideration the whole person, encompassing physical, emotional, mental, and spiritual dimensions. This model recognizes that health is not merely the absence of disease but a state of complete physical, mental, and social well-being. Here's an overview of the key components of the Holistic Nursing Model:

Holistic Assessment: The model begins with a comprehensive assessment of the patient that goes beyond physical symptoms. Nurses evaluate the patient's emotional state, mental health, spiritual beliefs, cultural background, and lifestyle factors. This holistic assessment helps in understanding the patient as a unique individual with diverse needs.

Individualized Care: Based on the assessment, holistic nursing care is tailored to meet the specific needs and preferences of each patient. There is no one-size-fits-all approach, as the model acknowledges that each person has their own unique healthcare journey.

Mind-Body-Spirit Connection: The model emphasizes the interconnectedness of the mind, body, and spirit. It recognizes that mental and emotional well-being can have a significant impact on physical health and vice versa. Therefore, nursing interventions address all these dimensions.

Patient-Centered Care: Holistic nursing places the patient at the center of care. It acknowledges the importance of the nurse-patient relationship and effective communication in providing the best care possible. Patients are active participants in their care decisions.

Complementary and Alternative Therapies: The model often incorporates complementary and alternative therapies (CAM), such as acupuncture, meditation, yoga, aromatherapy, and herbal medicine, when appropriate and acceptable to the patient. These therapies are used alongside conventional medical treatments.

Preventive Care: Holistic nursing places a strong emphasis on preventive care and health promotion. Nurses work with patients to identify risk factors and develop strategies for maintaining and improving overall wellness.

Cultural Competence: Cultural sensitivity is an essential aspect of the Holistic Nursing Model. Nurses respect and honor the cultural beliefs, values, and traditions of their patients, recognizing that these factors influence health and healing.

Promotion of Self-Care: Holistic nursing empowers patients to take an active role in their own care. Nurses educate patients about self-care practices and lifestyle choices that can enhance their well-being.

Ethical Practice: Ethical principles and values are integral to holistic nursing. Nurses navigate ethical dilemmas and decisions while upholding patient autonomy and respecting patients' wishes.

Holistic Healing Environment: The model acknowledges the importance of creating a healing environment that promotes relaxation, comfort, and a sense of security. This environment supports the patient's healing process.

Continuity of Care: Holistic nursing recognizes the value of continuity in care. Nurses aim to provide consistent care that follows the patient's healthcare journey, adapting interventions as needed.

The Holistic Nursing Model encourages nurses to see patients as whole beings and to provide care that addresses physical, emotional, mental, and spiritual aspects of health. It fosters a deep understanding of each patient's unique needs and beliefs, promoting not only the treatment of illness but also the cultivation of overall well-being. Holistic nursing aligns with the idea that healthcare should encompass the full spectrum of human existence and promote health and healing in the broadest sense.

The Importance of Mind-Body-Spirit Integration

The importance of mind-body-spirit integration in nursing cannot be overstated. This holistic approach recognizes that individuals are not just physical bodies with medical conditions but complex beings with interconnected dimensions. Here's a detailed explanation of why mind-body-spirit integration is crucial in nursing:

Comprehensive Care: Mind-body-spirit integration ensures that nurses consider all aspects of a patient's well-being. It goes beyond treating physical symptoms to address emotional, mental, and spiritual needs. This comprehensive care approach is essential for promoting holistic health.

Enhanced Healing: The mind and emotions play a significant role in the healing process. Stress, anxiety, and emotional distress can negatively impact physical health and recovery. Integrating mental and emotional support can enhance the patient's overall healing experience.

Psychosomatic Connection: There is a strong connection between the mind and the body, often referred to as the psychosomatic connection. Mental and emotional stress can manifest physically as symptoms or exacerbate existing medical conditions. Addressing mental and emotional well-being can alleviate physical suffering.

Promotion of Wellness: Mind-body-spirit integration is not limited to illness care but extends to wellness promotion. Nurses can educate patients about the importance of mental, emotional, and spiritual well-being in maintaining good health and preventing illness.

Holistic Assessment: Comprehensive patient assessments that consider the mind, body, and spirit provide a more accurate picture of a patient's health. This leads to better care planning and more effective interventions.

Prevention of Burnout: Nurses themselves can benefit from mind-body-spirit integration. The demands of nursing can be emotionally and mentally taxing. Integrating self-care practices, mindfulness, and stress reduction techniques can prevent burnout and support the nurse's own well-being.

Improved Coping Skills: Patients facing chronic illness, end-of-life issues, or emotional challenges benefit from strategies to cope with their circumstances. Mind-body-spirit integration equips nurses to provide patients with coping tools, resilience-building techniques, and emotional support.

Spiritual and Existential Support: Many patients grapple with spiritual and existential questions, especially during illness or near the end of life. Integrating spiritual and existential care helps patients find meaning, cope with existential concerns, and connect with their own belief systems for support.

Better Patient Outcomes: Research has shown that mind-body-spirit integration can lead to better patient outcomes, including improved pain management, reduced anxiety and depression, faster recovery times, and increased patient satisfaction.

Cultural Competence: Recognizing the importance of mind-body-spirit integration is essential in culturally competent care. Different cultures may have unique beliefs and practices related to the mind, body, and spirit. Nurses who are sensitive to these beliefs can provide more effective care.

Ethical Care: Ethical nursing practice includes respecting patients' autonomy and their wishes regarding their care. Mind-body-spirit integration ensures that nurses respect patients' values and beliefs, even if they differ from their own.

Mind-body-spirit integration in nursing acknowledges that true well-being encompasses physical, emotional, mental, and spiritual dimensions. This holistic approach fosters a deeper understanding of patients, supports their healing and well-being, and enhances the overall quality of care. It aligns with the idea that nursing is not just about treating diseases but about caring for the whole person in their journey toward health and healing.

Chapter 2:
The Holistic Assessment Process

Comprehensive Patient Assessment

Comprehensive patient assessment is a systematic and thorough process conducted by healthcare professionals, including nurses, to gather a holistic understanding of a patient's health status, needs, preferences, and potential risks. This assessment goes beyond addressing physical symptoms and involves considering the patient's emotional, mental, social, and spiritual dimensions. Here's a detailed explanation of comprehensive patient assessment:

Physical Assessment: This is the foundation of comprehensive assessment and involves evaluating the patient's physical health. It includes measuring vital signs (such as heart rate, blood pressure, temperature, and respiratory rate), conducting head-to-toe assessments, and assessing specific body systems relevant to the patient's condition.

Medical History: Gathering the patient's medical history involves obtaining information about their past illnesses, surgeries, allergies, chronic conditions, and medications. This historical data provides insights into the patient's health trajectory and helps identify potential risk factors.

Psychosocial Assessment: Nurses explore the patient's psychosocial well-being, including their emotional state, mental health, coping mechanisms, support systems, and stressors. This assessment helps identify emotional and mental health needs and informs interventions to address them.

Cultural and Spiritual Assessment: Recognizing the patient's cultural background and spiritual beliefs is essential for delivering culturally sensitive care. This assessment helps nurses understand how culture and spirituality influence the patient's perceptions of health and illness.

Nutritional Assessment: Evaluating the patient's dietary habits, nutritional intake, and hydration status is crucial for supporting their overall well-being. Nutritional assessments identify nutritional deficiencies or excesses that may impact the patient's health.

Functional Assessment: Assessing the patient's ability to perform daily activities and their level of independence provides insights into their functional status. This assessment is particularly relevant for elderly or chronically ill patients.

Pain Assessment: Evaluating the patient's pain experience, including its location, intensity, quality, and exacerbating/alleviating factors, helps guide pain management strategies.

Social Determinants of Health: Identifying social determinants of health, such as socioeconomic status, education level, housing conditions, and access to healthcare, helps nurses understand the broader context in which the patient lives and its impact on health.

Environmental Assessment: Evaluating the patient's living environment, including safety hazards and potential allergens, helps ensure a safe and supportive setting for recovery.

Risk Assessment: Identifying potential risks, such as fall risks, pressure ulcer risks, or risks for complications, enables nurses to implement preventive measures and interventions to mitigate these risks.

Communication and Collaboration: Comprehensive patient assessment involves effective communication with the patient, their families, and other members of the healthcare team. Collaboration ensures that all relevant information is considered and that the patient's needs are addressed comprehensively.

Documentation: Accurate and thorough documentation of the assessment findings is critical. Comprehensive documentation informs the care plan, facilitates communication among healthcare providers, and ensures continuity of care.

Comprehensive patient assessment forms the foundation for developing individualized care plans and making informed clinical decisions. It allows nurses to identify patient needs, plan appropriate interventions, and evaluate the effectiveness of interventions over time. By considering all dimensions of the patient's well-being, nurses can provide holistic care that addresses physical, emotional, mental, and spiritual aspects, ultimately promoting better patient outcomes and quality of life.

Assessing Physical Health

Assessing physical health is a fundamental component of comprehensive patient assessment in nursing and healthcare. It involves systematically gathering data and information about a patient's physical well-being to evaluate their overall health status and identify any potential health issues or concerns. Here's an explanation of assessing physical health:

Vital Signs Assessment: Vital signs are crucial indicators of a patient's physical health. Nurses routinely measure and monitor vital signs, including:

- Heart Rate (Pulse): Assessing the number of heartbeats per minute, which provides information about cardiovascular health and circulation.
- Blood Pressure: Measuring the force of blood against the arterial walls, which

helps identify hypertension or hypotension.

- Respiratory Rate: Counting the number of breaths per minute to assess lung and respiratory function.
- Temperature: Measuring body temperature to detect fever or hypothermia.
- Oxygen Saturation (SpO2): Assessing the amount of oxygen carried by hemoglobin in the blood, which indicates oxygenation status.

Physical Examination: A head-to-toe physical examination is conducted to assess the patient's overall physical condition. This includes examining various body systems, such as the:

- Cardiovascular System: Assessing the heart and blood vessels for abnormalities, murmurs, or irregular rhythms.

- Respiratory System: Listening to lung sounds and checking for signs of respiratory distress.
- Gastrointestinal System: Examining the abdomen for tenderness, masses, or organ enlargement.
- Musculoskeletal System: Evaluating the patient's mobility, strength, and joint function.
- Neurological System: Assessing mental status, cranial nerves, reflexes, and sensory function.
- Integumentary System: Inspecting the skin for lesions, rashes, wounds, or signs of infection.
- Genitourinary System: Examining the urinary system for signs of kidney or bladder issues.
- Eyes, Ears, Nose, and Throat (EENT): Checking the sensory organs for any abnormalities or deficits.

Pain Assessment: Assessing the patient's pain level is an essential component of physical health assessment. This includes determining the location, intensity, quality, duration, and aggravating or alleviating factors of pain. Understanding the patient's pain helps in effective pain management.

Functional Assessment: In addition to evaluating specific body systems, nurses may assess the patient's functional status. This involves assessing their ability to perform daily activities, including mobility, self-care, and activities of daily living (ADLs).

Nutritional Assessment: Evaluating the patient's nutritional status is essential for understanding their physical health. This includes assessing dietary habits, food allergies, nutritional intake, and hydration status. Malnutrition or dietary deficiencies can affect overall health.

Medication Review: Reviewing the patient's medication history helps assess their physical health. Nurses need to identify prescribed medications, over-the-counter drugs, and any potential interactions or adverse effects.

Laboratory and Diagnostic Tests: Depending on the patient's condition and clinical need, healthcare providers may order various laboratory tests, such as blood tests, imaging studies, or diagnostic procedures. The results of these tests provide valuable information about the patient's physical health and guide further assessment and treatment.

Health History: Gathering the patient's health history, including past medical conditions, surgeries, allergies, and family medical history, provides important context for assessing their current physical health.

Assessing physical health is a critical step in nursing care as it helps nurses and healthcare providers identify health problems, establish baseline data, and monitor changes in a patient's condition over time. This information guides the development of care plans, interventions, and treatments tailored to address the patient's specific physical health needs. Additionally, it forms an integral part of comprehensive patient assessment, which considers not only physical health but also emotional, mental, social, and spiritual aspects of a patient's well-being.

Assessing Emotional and Mental Well-being

Assessing emotional and mental well-being is a crucial aspect of comprehensive patient assessment in nursing and healthcare. It involves gathering information about a patient's emotional state, mental health, and psychological needs to understand their overall mental well-being and identify any potential concerns or issues. Here's an explanation of assessing emotional and mental well-being:

Establishing Rapport: Building trust and rapport with the patient is the first step in assessing emotional and mental well-being. Creating a safe and non-judgmental environment encourages patients to open up and share their thoughts and feelings.

Active Listening: Effective communication is essential for assessing emotional and mental well-being. Nurses practice active listening by giving their full attention, using open-ended questions, and providing empathetic responses to encourage patients to express their emotions and concerns.

Observation: Nurses observe patients' non-verbal cues, such as body language, facial expressions, and gestures, to gain insights into their emotional state. For example, signs of distress, agitation, sadness, or anxiety may be observed during the assessment.

Mental Status Examination (MSE): A mental status examination is a structured assessment that evaluates a patient's cognitive and emotional functioning. It includes assessing areas such as appearance, behavior, mood, thought process, thought content, perception, cognition, and insight.

Assessing Mood and Affect: Nurses ask patients about their current mood and emotions. Patients may describe their mood as sad, anxious, elated, or other emotions. Assessing affect involves evaluating their emotional expression during the conversation, such as flat affect or inappropriate emotional responses.

Assessing Thought Content: Nurses inquire about the content of the patient's thoughts. They assess whether the patient is experiencing any distressing or irrational thoughts, such as thoughts of self-harm or harm to others.

Suicidal and Homicidal Ideation: Assessing for suicidal or homicidal thoughts is critical in mental health assessments. Nurses ask direct questions to determine if the patient has thoughts of harming themselves or others and assess their intent and plan.

Psychosocial History: Gathering information about the patient's psychosocial history, including past mental health diagnoses, psychiatric hospitalizations, therapy or counseling, and medication history, provides important context for assessing current emotional and mental well-being.

Perception Assessment: Patients may report perceptual disturbances, such as hallucinations or delusions. Nurses inquire about any sensory experiences that may indicate altered perception.

Coping Strategies: Assessing the patient's coping mechanisms helps nurses understand how the patient deals with stressors and challenges. Effective coping strategies contribute to emotional resilience, while maladaptive strategies may indicate the need for intervention.

Support Systems: Evaluating the patient's support system, including family, friends, and community resources, provides insights into their social and emotional support network.

Screening Tools: Nurses may use validated screening tools and questionnaires to assess specific mental health conditions, such as depression, anxiety, or substance use disorders.

Cultural Competence: Recognizing and respecting cultural beliefs and values related to mental health is essential. Cultural competence ensures that the assessment process is sensitive to the patient's cultural background.

Patient Self-Report: Encouraging patients to self-report their emotional and mental well-being, including any symptoms or concerns they may have, is an important part of the assessment process.

Documentation: Thorough and accurate documentation of the assessment findings is critical. This information informs care planning, interventions, and ongoing monitoring of the patient's emotional and mental well-being.

Assessing emotional and mental well-being is essential for identifying mental health issues, emotional distress, or psychosocial factors that may impact a patient's overall health. It enables nurses to develop individualized care plans, provide appropriate interventions, and collaborate with mental health professionals when necessary to support the patient's emotional and mental well-being as part of holistic healthcare.

Assessing Spiritual and Existential Needs

Assessing spiritual and existential needs is an essential component of comprehensive patient assessment in nursing and healthcare. This assessment aims to understand a patient's spiritual beliefs, values, and existential concerns, recognizing that these aspects of well-being can significantly influence a patient's overall health and healing process. Here's an explanation of assessing spiritual and existential needs:

Establishing Trust and Respect: Building a trusting and respectful nurse-patient relationship is crucial when addressing spiritual and existential needs. Patients are more likely to share their beliefs and concerns when they feel safe and respected.

Assessment of Religious Beliefs: Nurses inquire about the patient's religious affiliation, beliefs, and practices. This includes asking about the patient's religious tradition, faith community, and how their religious beliefs influence their life and healthcare decisions.

Spiritual Beliefs and Values: Nurses assess the patient's personal spiritual beliefs and values, which may or may not align with a specific religious tradition. Patients may have unique spiritual perspectives that inform their understanding of life, illness, and healing.

Existential Concerns: Existential concerns often revolve around questions of purpose, meaning, suffering, life's challenges, and mortality. Nurses ask patients about any existential concerns they may have and explore how these concerns impact their overall well-being.

Spiritual Practices: Patients may engage in spiritual practices such as prayer, meditation, or rituals that provide them with comfort and strength. Nurses ask about these practices and how they contribute to the patient's sense of spirituality.

Crisis of Faith or Doubt: Some patients may experience crises of faith or periods of doubt in their beliefs, especially when facing serious illness or existential challenges. Nurses assess whether the patient is experiencing such crises and provide support as needed.

Cultural Competence: Recognizing and respecting cultural and religious diversity is crucial. Nurses should be sensitive to the cultural beliefs and practices related to spirituality and religion that may influence the patient's care.

Spiritual and Pastoral Care Resources: Nurses can collaborate with spiritual and pastoral care providers or chaplains to address the patient's spiritual and existential needs. These specialists can offer guidance, support, and spiritual care services tailored to the patient's beliefs and preferences.

Advance Directives and End-of-Life Preferences: Assessing the patient's advance directives and end-of-life preferences is essential, as these documents may reflect their spiritual and existential values, particularly regarding life-sustaining treatments and decision-making.

Assessing spiritual and existential needs is a patient-centered approach that recognizes the importance of these dimensions in a patient's life and healthcare journey. By addressing these needs, nurses and healthcare providers can offer support, promote emotional and mental well-being, and assist patients in finding meaning and comfort, particularly in times of illness, suffering, or end-of-life care.

This assessment contributes to the holistic care of the patient, recognizing them as a whole person with diverse dimensions of well-being.

Cultural Sensitivity in Assessment

Cultural sensitivity in assessment is the practice of recognizing and respecting the cultural beliefs, values, norms, and preferences of individuals and communities when conducting assessments in nursing and healthcare. It acknowledges that culture plays a significant role in shaping a person's health beliefs and behaviors, and it seeks to ensure that assessments are conducted in a culturally competent and respectful manner. Here's an explanation of the importance and key considerations for cultural sensitivity in assessment:

Importance of Cultural Sensitivity in Assessment

Respect for Diversity: Cultural sensitivity demonstrates respect for the diversity of patients and acknowledges that there is no one-size-fits-all approach to healthcare.

Accurate Assessment: Cultural sensitivity helps ensure that assessments are accurate and relevant. It prevents misinterpretation of cultural norms or beliefs as symptoms or issues.

Patient-Centered Care: Cultural sensitivity aligns with the principles of patient-centered care, where the patient's values, beliefs, and preferences are central to decision-making and care planning.

Key Considerations for Cultural Sensitivity in Assessment

Self-Awareness: Healthcare providers should engage in self-reflection to recognize their own cultural biases and assumptions. Being aware of one's cultural background and potential biases is the first step toward cultural sensitivity.

Respect for Beliefs: Nurses should respect and honor the cultural beliefs and practices of their patients. Avoid making judgments or assumptions about a patient's beliefs or practices.

Language and Communication: Assess the patient's language preferences and provide interpreters or translated materials when necessary. Ensure that communication is clear and culturally appropriate.

Non-Verbal Communication: Be aware of non-verbal cues and gestures that may have cultural significance. Avoid misinterpretation of body language.

Religious Beliefs: Assess the patient's religious beliefs and practices, particularly in the context of healthcare decisions, dietary restrictions, and end-of-life care preferences.

Family and Community: Understand the role of family and community in the patient's healthcare decisions. Some cultures prioritize collective decision-making rather than individual autonomy.

Modesty and Privacy: Respect cultural norms related to modesty and privacy. Ensure that assessments are conducted in a manner that respects the patient's comfort level.

Dietary Preferences: Be aware of dietary preferences and restrictions that may be based on cultural or religious beliefs. These may impact nutritional assessments and dietary recommendations.

Alternative Therapies: Some cultures use alternative or traditional healing practices alongside conventional medicine. Inquire about these practices and consider their potential impact on health.

Cultural Humility: Cultivate cultural humility, which involves ongoing learning and a willingness to adapt one's practice to be more culturally sensitive.

Cultural sensitivity in assessment is not only a professional responsibility but also a key element of providing quality, patient-centered care. It fosters mutual respect, trust, and effective communication between healthcare providers and patients from diverse cultural backgrounds, ultimately leading to improved healthcare outcomes and patient satisfaction.

Chapter 3:
Holistic Nursing Interventions

Holistic Care Planning

Holistic care planning is a comprehensive and patient-centered approach to healthcare that takes into consideration all aspects of an individual's well-being, including their physical, emotional, mental, social, and spiritual dimensions. The goal of holistic care planning is to develop a personalized care plan that addresses the unique needs, preferences, and goals of the patient. Here's an overview of the key components and principles of holistic care planning:

Comprehensive Assessment: Holistic care planning begins with a thorough and holistic assessment of the patient. This assessment includes evaluating the patient's physical health, emotional and mental well-being, social support systems, spiritual beliefs, cultural background, and any other factors that may influence their health and care.

Setting Goals: The care plan includes clear and specific goals that are developed in collaboration with the patient. These goals should be achievable, measurable, and aligned with the patient's desired outcomes.

Multidisciplinary Collaboration: Holistic care planning often involves collaboration among a team of healthcare professionals, including nurses, physicians, therapists, social workers, and spiritual care providers. Each team member contributes their expertise to address different aspects of the patient's well-being.

Integration of Services: The care plan integrates various services and interventions to address the patient's physical, emotional, mental, and social needs. This may include medical treatments, therapy, counseling, nutritional support, spiritual care, and social services.

Promotion of Self-Care: Holistic care planning empowers patients to take an active role in their own care. Patients are educated about self-care practices and strategies to maintain and improve their health and well-being.

Cultural Competence: Cultural sensitivity is essential in holistic care planning. The care plan should respect and incorporate the patient's cultural beliefs and practices, recognizing their impact on health and healing.

Spiritual and Existential Support: For patients with spiritual or existential concerns, the care plan may include support from chaplains or spiritual care providers to address these aspects of well-being.

Emotional and Psychological Support: Patients experiencing emotional or psychological challenges may receive counseling or therapy as part of the care plan. This support aims to improve mental health and emotional well-being.

Regular Evaluation and Adjustment: The care plan is not static; it evolves over time. Regular evaluations are conducted to assess progress toward goals and make necessary adjustments to the plan based on the patient's changing needs.

End-of-Life Planning: For patients with life-limiting illnesses or those in palliative care, holistic care planning may include discussions about end-of-life preferences, comfort measures, and support for both the patient and their family.

Documentation: Thorough and accurate documentation of the care plan, including goals, interventions, and outcomes, is essential for communication among healthcare providers and ensuring continuity of care.

Holistic care planning recognizes that health is a complex interplay of physical, emotional, mental, social, and spiritual factors. By addressing all these dimensions, healthcare providers can offer more comprehensive and effective care that promotes not only the treatment of illness but also the overall well-being and quality of life of the patient. It aligns with the principle that healthcare should focus on the whole person, not just the disease.

Integrating Alternative and Complementary Therapies

Integrating alternative and complementary therapies into healthcare involves incorporating non-conventional approaches alongside conventional medical treatments to address patients' health and well-being. These therapies can encompass a wide range of practices, such as acupuncture, herbal medicine, mindfulness meditation, yoga, aromatherapy, and more. The integration of these therapies acknowledges their potential benefits in promoting holistic health and healing. Here's an explanation of the key considerations and benefits of integrating alternative and complementary therapies:

Key Considerations for Integrating Alternative and Complementary Therapies:

Evidence-Based Approach: While some alternative and complementary therapies have shown promising results, it's important to prioritize evidence-based practices. Integrating therapies with proven effectiveness and safety ensures that patients receive beneficial interventions.

Collaborative Decision-Making: Informed shared decision-making involves discussing alternative therapies with patients, considering their preferences and goals, and collaboratively deciding on the best approach to care.

Healthcare Provider Education: Healthcare professionals should have a good understanding of alternative and complementary therapies to provide accurate information to patients and make informed recommendations.

Interdisciplinary Collaboration: Integrating these therapies often involves collaboration between different healthcare providers, such as nurses, physicians, and complementary therapy practitioners. Open communication is crucial to ensure coordinated and safe care.

Safety and Quality: Ensure that complementary therapy practitioners are licensed or certified, follow established safety guidelines, and adhere to ethical standards. Patient safety and quality of care are paramount.

Cultural and Religious Sensitivity: Different cultures and belief systems may have varying perspectives on alternative therapies. Cultural competence is essential in assessing patients' preferences and providing culturally sensitive care.

Potential Interactions: Be aware of potential interactions between alternative therapies and conventional treatments or medications. Some therapies may enhance or interfere with the effects of certain medications.

Benefits of Integrating Alternative and Complementary Therapies:

Holistic Approach: Integrating these therapies recognizes the interconnectedness of physical, emotional, mental, and spiritual dimensions of health, promoting a more holistic approach to patient care.

Enhanced Well-Being: Some therapies can contribute to stress reduction, relaxation, pain management, and improved quality of life. They may offer patients additional tools for managing their health challenges.

Individualized Care: Integrating these therapies allows for personalized care plans tailored to the patient's unique needs and preferences.

Reduced Side Effects: Some alternative therapies, when used in conjunction with conventional treatments, may help manage side effects of medical interventions.

Patient Empowerment: Integrating these therapies empowers patients to actively participate in their care and make informed decisions about their treatment options.

Cultural Sensitivity: For patients who value or have cultural ties to specific therapies, integration respects their cultural beliefs and practices.

Supportive Care: Complementary therapies can provide emotional and psychological support to patients undergoing medical treatments.

Preventive Care: Certain therapies emphasize preventive strategies and lifestyle modifications that promote overall wellness.

Integrating alternative and complementary therapies requires a balanced approach that considers patient preferences, clinical evidence, safety, and collaboration among healthcare providers. When integrated thoughtfully and ethically, these therapies can enhance patient-centered care, promoting a holistic approach that addresses both the physical and non-physical aspects of health and healing.

Promoting Mindfulness and Stress Reduction

Promoting mindfulness and stress reduction is a critical aspect of holistic healthcare and nursing practice. Mindfulness involves being fully present in the moment, paying attention to thoughts and feelings without judgment, and stress reduction techniques aim to alleviate the negative effects of stress on physical, emotional, and mental well-being. Here are some strategies and approaches for promoting mindfulness and stress reduction in nursing and healthcare:

Patient Education: Educate patients about the benefits of mindfulness and stress reduction techniques. Provide information on how these practices can improve their overall well-being and help manage various health conditions.

Mindfulness Meditation: Encourage patients to engage in mindfulness meditation. This practice involves focusing on the breath or a specific object while observing thoughts and feelings as they arise without attachment. Provide resources or refer patients to meditation classes or apps.

Deep Breathing Exercises: Teach patients deep breathing techniques, such as diaphragmatic breathing or the 4-7-8 technique, to help reduce stress and anxiety. These exercises can be performed anywhere and are effective in calming the nervous system.

Progressive Muscle Relaxation: Guide patients through progressive muscle relaxation exercises, where they systematically tense and then release muscle groups in the body. This practice helps reduce physical tension and stress.

Yoga and Tai Chi: Encourage patients to explore yoga or Tai Chi classes, which combine physical activity with mindfulness.

These practices improve flexibility, balance, and mental focus while promoting relaxation.

Journaling: Suggest patients keep a mindfulness journal to record their thoughts, emotions, and daily experiences. Reflecting on these entries can help increase self-awareness and reduce stress.

Nature and Outdoor Activities: Encourage patients to spend time in nature, go for walks, or engage in outdoor activities. Nature has a calming effect and can help reduce stress levels.

Stress Reduction Apps: Recommend mindfulness and stress reduction apps that offer guided meditation, breathing exercises, and relaxation techniques. These apps are accessible and can be used on smartphones or tablets.

Group Support: Facilitate or recommend support groups for patients dealing with similar stressors or health conditions. Group support can provide a sense of community and shared coping strategies.

Cognitive Behavioral Therapy (CBT): For patients with chronic stress or anxiety, consider referring them to CBT, a structured therapeutic approach that helps individuals identify and change negative thought patterns and behaviors.

Mindfulness-Based Stress Reduction (MBSR): MBSR programs are evidence-based interventions that combine mindfulness meditation and yoga. Patients can enroll in MBSR courses to learn and practice these techniques in a structured setting.

Self-Care Practices: Encourage patients to prioritize self-care by getting adequate sleep, maintaining a balanced diet, staying hydrated, and engaging in activities they enjoy.

Cultural Sensitivity: Be mindful of cultural preferences and beliefs related to stress reduction. Some patients may have cultural practices that promote relaxation, which should be respected and integrated into their care.

Regular Follow-Up: Follow up with patients to assess the effectiveness of mindfulness and stress reduction techniques. Adjust interventions as needed based on their feedback and progress.

Promoting mindfulness and stress reduction is not only beneficial for patients but also for healthcare providers. Nurses themselves can benefit from these practices to prevent burnout and enhance their own well-being, which, in turn, enables them to provide better care to their patients. By integrating these techniques into healthcare, nurses contribute to a holistic approach that addresses the emotional and mental well-being of patients and supports their overall health.

Nutrition and Holistic Wellness

Nutrition plays a central role in holistic wellness, as it directly impacts a person's physical, emotional, mental, and even spiritual well-being. A holistic approach to nutrition goes beyond simply providing nourishment; it considers the interconnectedness of various aspects of health. Here are key points regarding the relationship between nutrition and holistic wellness:

Physical Health: Nutrition is a cornerstone of physical well-being. A balanced diet provides essential nutrients, vitamins, and minerals necessary for optimal bodily functions. It supports the immune system, aids in maintaining a healthy weight, and contributes to overall vitality.

Emotional Well-Being: Diet can have a significant impact on mood and emotions. Nutrient-rich foods, such as those high in omega-3 fatty acids, antioxidants, and B vitamins, can help regulate mood and reduce the risk of depression and anxiety.

Mental Health: Proper nutrition is linked to cognitive function and mental clarity. A diet rich in antioxidants and healthy fats can support brain health and may reduce the risk of cognitive decline.

Energy Levels: Nutrient-dense foods provide sustained energy, helping individuals stay alert and focused throughout the day. Avoiding excessive sugar and processed foods can prevent energy crashes.

Digestive Health: A well-balanced diet that includes fiber-rich foods promotes a healthy digestive system. Digestive health is crucial for nutrient absorption and overall well-being.

Weight Management: Holistic nutrition focuses on achieving and maintaining a healthy weight through balanced eating habits rather than extreme diets. Sustainable weight management is essential for long-term wellness.

Chronic Disease Prevention: A nutritious diet is associated with a reduced risk of chronic diseases such as heart disease, diabetes, and certain cancers. It can also support management of these conditions in individuals who already have them.

Hydration: Proper hydration is a critical component of holistic wellness. Dehydration can lead to a range of health issues, including fatigue, headaches, and impaired cognitive function.

Stress Management: Some foods, such as those containing magnesium or antioxidants, can help the body manage stress. Additionally, mindful eating practices can reduce stress by promoting a positive relationship with food.

Cultural Sensitivity: Holistic nutrition respects cultural dietary preferences and traditions. It recognizes that cultural factors influence food choices and dietary practices.

Mindful Eating: Holistic nutrition encourages mindful eating, which involves being fully present during meals, savoring each bite, and listening to the body's hunger and fullness cues. This approach promotes a healthier relationship with food.

Spiritual Wellness: For some individuals, nutrition may be intertwined with their spiritual beliefs. Certain diets or food choices may align with their spiritual practices or values, contributing to a sense of spiritual well-being.

Holistic Assessment: Healthcare providers in a holistic approach assess not only a person's diet but also their lifestyle, stress levels, sleep patterns, and emotional relationship with food. These factors all influence nutritional choices and overall wellness.

Whole Foods: Holistic nutrition emphasizes whole, unprocessed foods. These foods are generally more nutrient-dense and provide a broader range of health benefits compared to heavily processed options.

Individualized Care: Holistic nutrition recognizes that one-size-fits-all dietary recommendations may not be suitable for everyone. It promotes individualized care, taking into account a person's unique needs, preferences, and goals.

Incorporating holistic nutrition into healthcare practice involves recognizing the interconnectedness of nutrition with physical, emotional, mental, and spiritual well-being. It emphasizes the importance of nourishing the whole person to support long-term health and wellness. Additionally, it encourages individuals to make mindful and sustainable dietary choices that align with their overall health goals.

Exercise and Physical Well-being

Promoting exercise and physical well-being is an integral part of patient care and health promotion. Nurses play a vital role in educating, encouraging, and supporting patients in adopting and maintaining a physically active lifestyle. Here's how exercise and physical well-being are addressed in nursing:

Assessment: Nurses assess patients' physical activity levels during initial assessments and throughout the patient's healthcare journey. They ask about exercise habits, limitations, and any barriers to physical activity. This assessment helps identify opportunities for intervention.

Education: Nurses provide patients with information about the benefits of regular exercise and physical activity. They explain how exercise can improve cardiovascular health, muscle strength, bone density, and mental well-being. Nurses also emphasize how exercise can help manage or prevent chronic conditions like diabetes and obesity.

Individualized Care: Nurses recognize that exercise recommendations should be individualized based on a patient's health status, age, fitness level, and personal preferences. They work with patients to develop exercise plans tailored to their specific needs and goals.

Safety Precautions: Nurses consider patient safety when recommending exercise. For patients with certain medical conditions or physical limitations, nurses ensure that exercise plans are safe and appropriate. They may collaborate with physical therapists or other specialists for guidance.

Medication Management: Nurses are aware of medications that can affect a patient's exercise capacity or response to physical activity. They monitor for any side effects or interactions that may impact a patient's ability to exercise safely.

Motivation and Support: Nurses provide motivation and support to encourage patients to adhere to their exercise routines. They may use motivational interviewing techniques to explore patients' readiness for change and help them set achievable goals.

Monitoring Progress: Nurses track patients' progress in terms of physical fitness and overall well-being. They document changes in exercise tolerance, weight, and other relevant health indicators. This information guides care planning and adjustments to exercise regimens.

Patient Education Materials: Nurses may provide patients with educational materials on exercise, including guidelines, resources, and tips for staying active. These materials reinforce the importance of physical well-being.

Behavioral Counseling: Nurses may offer behavioral counseling to help patients overcome barriers to exercise, such as lack of motivation, time constraints, or fears of injury. They assist patients in developing strategies for incorporating exercise into their daily routines.

Holistic Approach: Nurses consider exercise as part of a holistic approach to health and wellness. They recognize the interconnectedness of physical, emotional, and mental well-being and address exercise in this context.

Collaboration: Nurses collaborate with other healthcare professionals, such as physical therapists, occupational therapists, and exercise physiologists, to provide comprehensive care plans for patients with complex exercise needs.

Cultural Competence: Nurses are culturally sensitive when discussing exercise and physical well-being, recognizing that cultural beliefs and practices can influence a person's approach to exercise.

By integrating exercise promotion and physical well-being into nursing practice, healthcare providers contribute to the prevention of chronic diseases, enhancement of patient outcomes, and overall improvement of patients' quality of life. Nurses serve as advocates and educators, empowering individuals to take an active role in their health and well-being through regular physical activity.

The Role of Holistic Nursing in Pain Management

Holistic nursing plays a significant role in pain management by addressing pain from a comprehensive perspective, considering not only the physical aspect but also the emotional, mental, social, and spiritual dimensions of pain. Holistic nurses prioritize patient-centered care, which aims to alleviate pain and enhance the overall well-being of individuals. Here's how holistic nursing contributes to effective pain management:

Comprehensive Pain Assessment: Holistic nurses conduct a thorough pain assessment that goes beyond the physical aspects of pain. They inquire about the patient's emotional state, stress levels, coping mechanisms, and any spiritual or existential concerns that may impact pain perception.

Patient-Centered Approach: Holistic nursing places the patient at the center of care. Nurses work collaboratively with patients to develop individualized pain management plans that align with the patient's goals, values, and preferences.

Pain Education: Nurses educate patients about the nature of pain, its potential causes, and available pain management strategies. This education fosters a better understanding of pain and empowers patients to actively participate in their pain management.

Non-Pharmacological Interventions: Holistic nurses integrate non-pharmacological pain management interventions, such as relaxation techniques, guided imagery, mindfulness, music therapy, and massage, into the care plan. These approaches can help alleviate pain and reduce the need for medications.

Pharmacological Management: Holistic nurses collaborate with healthcare providers to ensure that pain medications are prescribed appropriately and that potential side effects or interactions are monitored. They also educate patients about the safe use of pain medications.

Emotional Support: Holistic nurses offer emotional support to patients experiencing pain. They create a compassionate and empathetic environment where patients feel comfortable expressing their emotional responses to pain, including fear, anxiety, or frustration.

Mind-Body Connection: Holistic nursing recognizes the mind-body connection and the impact of stress on pain perception. Nurses help patients manage stress through relaxation techniques, deep breathing exercises, and other stress-reduction strategies.

Spiritual and Existential Care: For patients with spiritual or existential concerns related to pain, holistic nurses may involve chaplains or spiritual care providers to provide support and guidance in addressing these dimensions of pain.

Cultural Sensitivity: Holistic nurses are culturally sensitive to patients' beliefs and practices related to pain and pain management. They respect cultural preferences for specific treatments or rituals that may provide comfort.

Holistic Assessment Tools: Nurses may use holistic assessment tools to evaluate the patient's overall well-being and the impact of pain on different aspects of their life. These tools help identify areas where additional support may be needed.

Interdisciplinary Collaboration: Holistic nurses collaborate with a multidisciplinary team, including physicians, physical therapists, psychologists, and others, to provide comprehensive pain management. This collaborative approach addresses pain from multiple angles.

Empowerment: Holistic nursing empowers patients to take an active role in their pain management. Patients are encouraged to communicate their pain levels, preferences, and concerns openly, fostering a sense of control over their pain.

Incorporating a holistic approach to pain management recognizes that pain is a complex and individualized experience. By addressing pain holistically, nurses aim to not only alleviate physical discomfort but also promote emotional well-being, enhance coping skills, and support patients in their journey toward improved quality of life.

Chapter 4: Nurturing Emotional and Mental Health

The Nurse's Role in Mental Health

The nurse's role in mental health care is multifaceted and crucial in providing comprehensive, compassionate, and effective support to individuals experiencing mental health challenges. Mental health nursing encompasses a wide range of responsibilities that focus on promoting mental well-being, preventing mental illness, and assisting individuals in their recovery journey. Here are key aspects of the nurse's role in mental health:

Assessment: Mental health nurses conduct thorough assessments to evaluate patients' mental and emotional states. They use standardized assessment tools, clinical interviews, and observations to identify mental health disorders, symptoms, risk factors, and strengths.

Diagnosis: Based on assessments, mental health nurses collaborate with other healthcare professionals to formulate accurate diagnoses. These diagnoses guide treatment planning and interventions.

Treatment Planning: Nurses work with the healthcare team and patients to develop individualized treatment plans that may include medication management, therapy, counseling, and psychosocial interventions. They consider patients' preferences and cultural factors in treatment planning.

Medication Management: Mental health nurses often administer and monitor psychiatric medications. They educate patients about their medications, potential side effects, and the importance of adherence. Medication management is done in collaboration with psychiatrists or other prescribers.

Therapeutic Relationships: Establishing and maintaining therapeutic relationships with patients is a cornerstone of mental health nursing. Nurses offer emotional support, empathy, and a nonjudgmental attitude to build trust and rapport with patients.

Crisis Intervention: In times of crisis or acute distress, mental health nurses provide immediate support and intervention. They assess for safety, facilitate de-escalation, and coordinate emergency services when needed.

Education: Mental health nurses educate patients and their families about mental health conditions, treatment options, coping strategies, and relapse prevention. They promote mental health literacy to reduce stigma and increase understanding.

Advocacy: Nurses advocate for patients' rights and access to appropriate care. They ensure that patients are treated with dignity and respect and that their voices are heard in treatment decisions.

Group Therapy: Many mental health nurses lead or facilitate group therapy sessions. These group settings provide a supportive environment for patients to share experiences, learn from one another, and develop coping skills.

Family Support: Nurses involve patients' families in the treatment process when appropriate. They provide education to families on how to support their loved ones and navigate the challenges of mental illness.

Prevention and Health Promotion: Mental health nurses engage in preventive efforts to reduce the risk of mental health issues. This may involve community outreach, awareness campaigns, and education on stress management and mental well-being.

Rehabilitation and Recovery: For individuals with chronic mental health conditions, nurses play a key role in rehabilitation and recovery support. They help patients set achievable goals, learn life skills, and reintegrate into the community.

Self-Care and Burnout Prevention: Mental health nursing can be emotionally demanding. Nurses prioritize self-care to maintain their own mental well-being and prevent burnout. They seek support and supervision when needed.

Continuing Education: Staying up-to-date with advances in mental health care and evidence-based practices is essential for mental health nurses. They engage in ongoing education and training to enhance their knowledge and skills.

Advocacy for Mental Health Policy: Some mental health nurses engage in policy advocacy to promote improvements in mental healthcare delivery, access, and funding.

The nurse's role in mental health is critical in providing holistic care that addresses not only the symptoms of mental illness but also the emotional, social, and cultural aspects of an individual's life. By fostering therapeutic relationships, promoting recovery, and advocating for patients' well-being, mental health nurses contribute significantly to improving the mental health of individuals and communities.

Building Therapeutic Relationships

Building therapeutic relationships is a foundational aspect of nursing practice, as it establishes trust, rapport, and effective communication between nurses and patients.

These relationships are essential for providing high-quality care and supporting patients' physical, emotional, and psychological well-being. Here are key principles and strategies for building therapeutic relationships:

Establish Trust: Trust is the cornerstone of any therapeutic relationship. Nurses must be reliable, honest, and consistent in their interactions with patients. Building trust takes time and requires a commitment to confidentiality and respect for patients' autonomy.

Empathy: Empathy is the ability to understand and share in the emotions of another person. Express empathy by acknowledging patients' feelings, using empathetic statements, and demonstrating compassion. Patients need to know that their emotions are recognized and validated.

Respect: Treat each patient with dignity and respect. Use appropriate titles, ask for their preferences regarding how they'd like to be addressed, and respect their cultural and religious beliefs. Always maintain confidentiality.

Cultural Competence: Recognize and appreciate cultural diversity. Be sensitive to cultural practices, beliefs, and values that may influence patients' healthcare decisions. Cultural competence fosters trust and understanding.

Nonverbal Communication: Pay attention to your nonverbal cues, including body language, tone of voice, and facial expressions. Ensure that your nonverbal signals are consistent with your verbal messages.

Effective Communication: Use clear, concise, and simple language when communicating with patients. Avoid medical jargon and provide explanations in a way that patients can easily understand. Encourage questions and provide written materials when appropriate.

Boundaries: Maintain professional boundaries with patients. Avoid self-disclosure of personal information unless it serves a therapeutic purpose. Be aware of potential boundary violations and address them promptly.

Empowerment: Empower patients by involving them in their care plans and helping them make informed decisions about their health. Encourage self-care and offer resources for patients to learn more about their conditions.

Conflict Resolution: Address conflicts or disagreements in a constructive manner. Be open to discussing concerns and work toward resolution collaboratively. Seek assistance from colleagues or supervisors when needed.

Consistency: Be consistent in your care and interactions with patients. Patients appreciate knowing what to expect and feeling that their care is stable and dependable.

Follow-Up: Maintain continuity of care by following up with patients as needed. Check in on their progress, address any concerns or questions, and ensure that they have the support they need.

Self-Care: Practicing self-care is essential for nurses. Managing your own stress and emotional well-being allows you to be present and attentive to patients without becoming emotionally drained.

Building therapeutic relationships is a dynamic process that evolves over time. It requires ongoing effort, empathy, and a commitment to providing patient-centered care. These relationships not only enhance the patient experience but also contribute to improved clinical outcomes and overall patient satisfaction.

Techniques for Emotional Support

Providing emotional support is a fundamental aspect of nursing care, as it helps patients cope with the emotional challenges that often accompany illness, hospitalization, or medical procedures. Nurses play a crucial role in offering comfort, reassurance, and empathy to patients and their families. Here are some techniques for providing emotional support in nursing:

Validation: Validate patients' feelings and experiences. Let them know that their emotions are normal responses to challenging situations. For example, you might say, "It's okay to feel scared or anxious; many patients do."

Supportive Touch: Offer appropriate physical touch, such as holding a patient's hand, providing a comforting pat on the shoulder, or giving a gentle hug when appropriate. Touch can convey warmth and compassion.

Use of Therapeutic Communication: Employ therapeutic communication techniques, such as open-ended questions, reflection, and paraphrasing, to facilitate meaningful conversations. Encourage patients to share their concerns and fears.

Privacy and Confidentiality: Ensure that conversations about emotional issues are conducted in private to protect patients' confidentiality and dignity. Patients may feel more comfortable discussing sensitive matters in a private setting.

Emotional Presence: Be emotionally present with patients. Avoid multitasking or appearing rushed during interactions. Show that you are fully engaged and available to provide support.

Patient Education: Provide information and education to help patients better understand their conditions and treatment options. Knowledge can alleviate anxiety and empower patients to make informed decisions.

Create a Comforting Environment: Make the patient's environment as comforting as possible. Adjust lighting, temperature, and noise levels to promote relaxation. Offer a warm blanket or soothing music, if appropriate.

Offer Reassurance: Reassure patients that they are not alone in their journey. Let them know that the healthcare team is dedicated to providing the best care possible and that their well-being is a top priority.

Encourage Expression of Feelings: Encourage patients to express their feelings through creative outlets like journaling, drawing, or talking to a therapist or counselor. Expressing emotions can be therapeutic.

Provide Emotional Resources: Offer information about support groups, counseling services, or other resources available to help patients and their families cope with emotional distress.

Normalize Emotions: Normalize the emotional responses patients may be experiencing. Explain that it's common to feel a range of emotions during illness or recovery, including fear, anger, sadness, and frustration.

Respect Cultural and Spiritual Beliefs: Be sensitive to patients' cultural and spiritual beliefs, as these can influence how they cope with illness and express emotions. Respect their practices and offer appropriate spiritual or cultural support.

Self-Care: Don't forget to practice self-care to manage your own emotional well-being. Caring for patients who are experiencing emotional distress can be emotionally challenging, so seek support from colleagues or supervisors when needed.

Providing emotional support requires empathy, active listening, and a compassionate approach. By offering emotional support, nurses not only enhance the patient experience but also contribute to better emotional and psychological outcomes for patients and their families.

Addressing Anxiety and Depression Holistically

Addressing anxiety and depression holistically in nursing involves a comprehensive approach that considers the physical, emotional, mental, social, and spiritual aspects of the patient's well-being. Nurses play a vital role in providing holistic care to individuals experiencing these mental health challenges. Here are strategies for addressing anxiety and depression holistically:

Assessment: Conduct a thorough assessment to understand the patient's mental health history, current symptoms, and any contributing factors. This assessment should include a review of physical health, medication use, and psychosocial stressors.

Medication Management: If medication is part of the treatment plan, provide education about the prescribed medications, potential side effects, and the importance of adherence. Monitor for medication effectiveness and side effects, and report any concerns to the healthcare team.

Psychotherapy: Encourage patients to engage in psychotherapy or counseling, such as cognitive-behavioral therapy (CBT) or interpersonal therapy. These evidence-based approaches can help patients manage symptoms and improve coping skills.

Supportive Relationships: Build therapeutic relationships with patients based on trust, empathy, and active listening. Provide emotional support, reassurance, and encouragement to help patients feel understood and valued.

Stress Reduction Techniques: Teach patients stress reduction techniques, such as mindfulness meditation, deep breathing exercises, progressive muscle relaxation, or yoga. These practices can help manage symptoms and reduce stress.

Nutrition: Promote a balanced diet rich in nutrients, as diet can influence mental health. Encourage patients to reduce the consumption of processed foods and sugars, which can negatively affect mood.

Sleep Hygiene: Provide guidance on sleep hygiene to help patients improve their sleep patterns. Lack of sleep can exacerbate symptoms of anxiety and depression.

Social Support: Encourage patients to engage with their support network, whether it's family, friends, or support groups. Social connections can provide emotional support and reduce feelings of isolation.

Cultural Competence: Be culturally sensitive and respectful of patients' cultural beliefs and practices. Recognize how culture may influence the expression and management of anxiety and depression.

Spiritual Support: For patients with spiritual beliefs, provide opportunities for spiritual support through chaplaincy services or discussions with the healthcare team.

Spiritual beliefs can be a source of comfort and coping.

Self-Care Promotion: Help patients develop self-care routines that prioritize their physical, emotional, and mental well-being. Encourage activities that bring joy and a sense of purpose.

Follow-Up and Monitoring: Continuously assess and monitor the patient's progress and response to treatment. Adjust the care plan as needed to ensure it remains effective.

By addressing anxiety and depression holistically, nurses contribute to better outcomes for patients, promoting not only symptom relief but also overall well-being and quality of life. The holistic approach recognizes that mental health is interconnected with physical, emotional, social, and spiritual dimensions, and that each aspect must be considered in the care of individuals with anxiety and depression.

Trauma-Informed Care

Trauma-informed care (TIC) in nursing is an approach that recognizes the widespread impact of trauma on individuals and integrates this understanding into nursing practice. It emphasizes creating a safe and supportive healthcare environment that fosters trust, empowerment, and healing for patients who have experienced trauma. Here are key principles and practices of trauma-informed care:

Awareness and Understanding: Nurses should be educated about the prevalence and effects of trauma, including adverse childhood experiences (ACEs) and other forms of trauma, such as military trauma or interpersonal violence. Understanding the potential triggers and symptoms of trauma is essential.

Safety: Create a physically and emotionally safe healthcare environment. Ensure that patients feel secure during their interactions with healthcare providers. Use non-threatening language, maintain privacy, and consider the physical layout of the healthcare facility.

Trustworthiness and Transparency: Be honest and transparent in your communication with patients. Build trust by following through on promises, respecting boundaries, and providing clear information about procedures, diagnoses, and treatment options.

Empowerment and Choice: Involve patients in their care and treatment decisions. Offer choices whenever possible, giving patients a sense of control over their healthcare. Recognize that individuals who have experienced trauma may feel disempowered and work to restore their sense of agency.

Cultural Sensitivity: Be culturally competent and respectful of patients' backgrounds, beliefs, and values. Trauma-informed care should be sensitive to cultural diversity.

Trauma Screening: Use trauma-informed screening tools to assess patients for a history of trauma. These screenings can help identify patients who may benefit from additional support or interventions.

Avoiding Retraumatization: Be mindful of language, behaviors, and procedures that may inadvertently trigger or re-traumatize patients. Avoid making assumptions or judgments about their experiences.

Individualized Care Plans: Develop individualized care plans that take into account the patient's trauma history and any triggers or specific needs they may have. Address trauma-related symptoms and incorporate trauma-sensitive interventions.

Self-Care for Nurses: Nurses should also practice self-care and seek support when dealing with patients who have experienced trauma. Hearing traumatic stories can be emotionally challenging, and nurses must manage their own well-being to provide effective care.

Trauma-informed care recognizes that trauma can have a lasting impact on a person's physical and emotional health. By implementing these principles and practices, nurses can help create a healthcare environment that promotes healing, resilience, and recovery for patients who have experienced trauma.

Chapter 5:
Fostering Spiritual and Existential Health

Spirituality in Healthcare

Spirituality in healthcare refers to the recognition and integration of spiritual beliefs, values, and practices into the provision of healthcare services. It recognizes that spirituality is an important aspect of holistic well-being and that it can significantly impact an individual's health and healing process. Here are key aspects of spirituality in healthcare:

Recognition of Spirituality: Healthcare providers acknowledge that spirituality is an integral part of the human experience and that it plays a significant role in the overall health and well-being of individuals.

Respect for Diversity: Spirituality in healthcare recognizes and respects the diversity of spiritual beliefs and practices among individuals. It is inclusive of various religious traditions as well as secular and non-religious spiritual perspectives.

Holistic Care: Spirituality is viewed as one of the dimensions of holistic care, alongside physical, emotional, mental, and social well-being. Healthcare providers consider the whole person, addressing physical, emotional, and spiritual needs.

Open and Non-Judgmental Communication: Healthcare providers engage in open, non-judgmental, and empathetic communication with patients about their spiritual concerns and beliefs. Patients are encouraged to express their spirituality freely.

Supporting Spiritual Practices: Healthcare facilities may provide space and resources for patients to engage in spiritual practices, such as prayer, meditation, or reflection. This supports patients in maintaining their spiritual routines during hospitalization.

Cultural Competence: Healthcare providers are culturally competent and sensitive to the spiritual beliefs and practices of diverse patient populations. They respect cultural rituals and preferences related to healthcare.

Ethical Considerations: Ethical considerations related to spirituality, such as respecting patients' autonomy and religious preferences, are upheld in healthcare decision-making.

Research and Education: Spirituality in healthcare is an area of ongoing research and education. Healthcare professionals stay informed about best practices and emerging research related to spirituality and health.

Self-Care for Healthcare Providers: Healthcare providers must practice self-care to address their own spiritual and emotional needs. Caring for patients' spiritual well-being can be emotionally challenging, and self-care is crucial for maintaining provider well-being.

Spirituality in healthcare recognizes that the mind, body, and spirit are interconnected, and that addressing spiritual needs can contribute to improved health outcomes and a sense of well-being for patients. It supports a patient-centered approach that respects and integrates the spiritual dimension of each individual's life.

Coping with Existential Questions

Coping with existential questions in nursing involves providing support and guidance to patients who are grappling with profound questions about the meaning and purpose of life, especially in the context of illness, suffering, or the end of life. These questions often touch on the spiritual and philosophical aspects of existence and can be deeply challenging for patients. Here are some strategies for nurses to help patients cope with existential questions:

Active Listening: Create a safe and non-judgmental space for patients to express their existential concerns. Listen attentively to their thoughts, fears, and questions without interrupting or rushing the conversation.

Validation: Validate patients' feelings and existential questions as normal and meaningful. Let them know that it's common to reflect on these issues, especially during times of illness or crisis.

Open-Ended Questions: Encourage patients to share their thoughts and feelings by asking open-ended questions. For example, you can ask, "Can you tell me more about what's on your mind?" or "What do you find most meaningful in your life?"

Reflective Exploration: Engage in reflective conversations with patients. Ask thought-provoking questions like, "What gives your life meaning?" or "What are your hopes and fears about the future?"

Empathetic Responses: Respond with empathy and compassion to patients' existential concerns. Offer statements like, "I can see that this is a deeply important issue for you," or "I'm here to support you as you explore these questions."

Respect for Beliefs: Respect and honor patients' spiritual and philosophical beliefs, even if they differ from your own. Avoid imposing your beliefs on them and maintain an open and non-judgmental attitude.

Spiritual and Religious Resources: Connect patients with spiritual leaders, chaplains, or religious counselors who can provide guidance and support in addressing existential questions from a faith-based perspective.

Support Groups: Inform patients about support groups or therapy options where they can explore existential questions with others who may be facing similar concerns.

Cultural Sensitivity: Be culturally sensitive to patients' beliefs and practices related to existential questions. Recognize the influence of culture on how patients approach these issues.

Encourage Self-Reflection: Encourage patients to engage in self-reflection through journaling, meditation, or other contemplative practices. These activities can help patients explore their thoughts and feelings more deeply.

Narrative Medicine: Incorporate narrative medicine techniques, such as storytelling and reflective writing, to help patients make sense of their experiences and create a coherent narrative of their lives.

Support for Advance Care Planning: Assist patients in documenting their preferences for end-of-life care through advance care directives. These discussions can help patients address existential questions related to death and dying.

Interdisciplinary Collaboration: Collaborate with other members of the healthcare team, including social workers, psychologists, and spiritual counselors, to provide comprehensive support for patients' existential concerns.

Self-Care for Nurses: Caring for patients who are grappling with existential questions can be emotionally challenging. Nurses should practice self-care and seek support from colleagues or supervisors when needed.

Coping with existential questions requires a compassionate and patient-centered approach that honors the unique journey of each individual. By providing support and guidance in addressing these profound questions, nurses can help patients find meaning and purpose in their lives, even in the face of illness or adversity.

End-of-Life Spiritual Care

End-of-life spiritual care is a compassionate approach to providing care and support to individuals who are facing the end of their lives. It recognizes the significance of addressing spiritual and existential needs during this critical time.

For example, imagine a terminally ill patient who is reflecting on their life and grappling with profound questions about the meaning and purpose of their existence. They may be feeling anxious, fearful, or uncertain about what lies ahead. End-of-life spiritual care involves actively listening to this patient's concerns, offering a non-judgmental and empathetic presence, and encouraging them to express their thoughts and emotions. By providing a safe space for such conversations, healthcare providers help the patient explore their existential concerns and find a sense of peace and understanding.

Additionally, consider a family who is at the bedside of a loved one who is dying. The family may have specific spiritual or religious traditions that they wish to observe during this time, such as saying prayers or performing rituals. End-of-life spiritual care involves respecting and accommodating these practices, ensuring that the family's spiritual needs are met, and facilitating a meaningful and sacred experience.

Furthermore, end-of-life spiritual care may involve collaboration with a chaplain or spiritual counselor who can provide specialized support based on the patient's faith tradition. For instance, if a patient is a devout member of a particular religious community, the chaplain can offer prayers, readings, or sacraments that align with that tradition, bringing comfort and solace to the patient and their family.

Ultimately, end-of-life spiritual care aims to address the profound questions, fears, and spiritual needs that individuals and their families may encounter during the dying process. It honors diversity, respects individual beliefs, and provides emotional support, helping patients and families find meaning and connection during this deeply personal and challenging phase of life.

Spiritual Self-Care for Nurses

Spiritual self-care for nurses refers to the intentional practices and activities that nurses engage in to nurture their spiritual well-being and maintain a sense of meaning, purpose, and inner peace in their lives. It recognizes that nursing is a demanding and emotionally taxing profession, and spiritual self-care is a way for nurses to cope with the challenges they encounter and sustain their emotional and psychological resilience.

Spiritual self-care for nurses can encompass a wide range of practices and beliefs, and it's highly individualized, reflecting each nurse's personal spirituality. Some common components of spiritual self-care for nurses include:

Meditation and Mindfulness: Engaging in meditation or mindfulness exercises to center oneself, reduce stress, and stay present in the moment.

Prayer and Spiritual Rituals: If a nurse has religious beliefs, they may engage in prayer or participate in spiritual rituals that align with their faith.

Reflection and Journaling: Taking time for self-reflection, contemplation, and journaling to explore one's values, beliefs, and the deeper meaning of their work.

Nature Connection: Spending time in nature to find solace, rejuvenation, and spiritual inspiration.

Yoga or Tai Chi: Practicing physical activities that promote relaxation, self-awareness, and a sense of spiritual connection.

Reading and Study: Engaging with spiritual or philosophical literature to expand one's understanding of spirituality and personal growth.

Community Involvement: Participating in spiritual or community groups that provide a sense of belonging and support.

Creative Expression: Using art, music, writing, or other creative outlets to express one's spirituality and emotions.

Volunteer Work: Engaging in acts of service to give back to the community and find spiritual fulfillment.

Gratitude Practice: Cultivating gratitude by regularly acknowledging and appreciating the positive aspects of life and work.

Boundaries: Setting boundaries to ensure a healthy work-life balance and create space for spiritual practices.

Self-Compassion: Treating oneself with kindness and self-compassion, recognizing that self-care is essential for well-being.

Support: Seeking support from spiritual leaders, counselors, or therapists when dealing with spiritual or existential questions.

Colleague Connections: Sharing spiritual experiences and self-care practices with colleagues to create a supportive workplace culture.

Continued Learning: Pursuing educational opportunities to deepen one's spiritual knowledge and personal growth.

Spiritual self-care acknowledges that nurses' well-being extends beyond physical and emotional aspects and includes their spiritual dimension. By incorporating spiritual self-care practices into their lives, nurses can find balance, meaning, and resilience in their demanding profession.

Chapter 6:
Holistic Nursing in Special Populations

Holistic Care for Pediatric Patients

Holistic care for pediatric patients is an approach to healthcare that recognizes the interconnectedness of a child's physical, emotional, social, and spiritual well-being. It considers the whole child, including their unique needs, preferences, and developmental stage, to provide comprehensive and patient-centered care. Here's an explanation of holistic care for pediatric patients:

Physical Health: Holistic care encompasses the child's physical health, including preventive care, diagnosis, and treatment of illnesses or conditions. It focuses on promoting optimal growth and development, nutrition, and physical activity.

Emotional and Mental Well-being: Holistic care acknowledges the importance of emotional and mental health in children. It addresses emotional challenges, such as anxiety, depression, and behavioral issues, by providing counseling, therapy, or interventions tailored to the child's age and developmental level.

Social Needs: Pediatric patients often have social needs related to family dynamics, peer interactions, and community involvement. Holistic care considers these factors and may involve social workers or support groups to address social challenges and promote healthy relationships.

Spiritual and Existential Needs: While spirituality may not have religious connotations for all children, it can encompass questions about meaning, purpose, and connection. Holistic care respects and addresses these spiritual and existential aspects, providing guidance and support as needed.

Cultural Sensitivity: Holistic care is culturally sensitive, recognizing the diversity of patients' backgrounds, beliefs, and values. It respects cultural traditions and customs in healthcare decision-making and treatment plans.

Family-Centered Care: Holistic care includes the family as an integral part of the child's care team. It recognizes the family's role in the child's well-being and involves them in care planning and decision-making.

Preventive Care: Holistic care emphasizes preventive healthcare, including vaccinations, screenings, and health education, to maintain the child's well-being and detect potential issues early.

Developmental Assessment: Holistic care includes developmental assessments to monitor a child's physical, cognitive, emotional, and social development. This helps identify any developmental delays or concerns.

Individualized Care Plans: Care plans are individualized to meet each child's specific needs and preferences. They consider the child's developmental stage, health history, and family context.

Pain and Symptom Management: For children experiencing pain or symptoms, holistic care focuses on effective pain management and symptom relief while addressing the emotional and psychological aspects of suffering.

Educational Support: For school-age children, holistic care may involve collaborating with educators and providing resources to support their academic success and overall development.

Play and Creative Therapies: Play therapy, art therapy, and other creative therapies are often used in pediatric holistic care to help children express their emotions, cope with stress, and process their experiences.

Emotional Support for Families: Pediatric holistic care recognizes the emotional impact of a child's illness on the entire family. Support and counseling are provided to parents and caregivers to help them navigate these challenges.

In essence, holistic care for pediatric patients acknowledges that a child's well-being is influenced by various interconnected factors. It aims to provide comprehensive, patient-centered care that addresses the physical, emotional, social, and spiritual dimensions of a child's health, fostering overall growth and development.

Caring for the Elderly Holistically

Caring for the elderly holistically in nursing involves a comprehensive and patient-centered approach that considers the physical, emotional, social, and spiritual aspects of their well-being. As individuals age, they often face a range of health challenges, and holistic nursing care aims to address these challenges while promoting overall quality of life and independence. Here's an explanation of how holistic care is applied to elderly patients:

Caregiver Support: Recognizing the role of family caregivers, holistic care also involves providing support and education to family members who play a crucial role in the care of elderly patients.

Physical Health: Holistic care for the elderly begins with assessing and addressing their physical health needs. This includes managing chronic conditions, monitoring vital signs, and ensuring proper nutrition and hydration. Falls prevention, medication management, and pain management are also essential components.

Emotional Well-being: Recognizing the emotional needs of elderly patients is crucial. Many elderly individuals may experience feelings of loneliness, anxiety, or depression. Holistic nursing care involves providing emotional support, active listening, and interventions such as cognitive-behavioral therapy or counseling when necessary.

Social Engagement: Social isolation is a common issue among the elderly. Holistic care focuses on promoting social engagement and a sense of belonging. Activities, social groups, and family involvement are encouraged to combat loneliness and depression.

Cognitive Health: Addressing cognitive health is vital, especially in cases of dementia or cognitive decline. Holistic care includes cognitive stimulation activities, memory care programs, and support for both patients and their families in coping with cognitive changes.

Spiritual and Existential Support: Holistic nursing acknowledges the importance of spirituality and existential concerns among the elderly. Providing opportunities for spiritual expression, such as visits from chaplains or participation in religious activities, can be part of holistic care.

Pain Management: Managing pain effectively is essential for elderly patients. Holistic care involves assessing pain levels, using a combination of pharmacological and non-pharmacological interventions, and addressing the emotional impact of pain.

Nutrition and Hydration: Ensuring that elderly patients receive proper nutrition and hydration is fundamental to their well-being.

Holistic care includes nutritional assessments, dietary adjustments, and monitoring for dehydration or malnutrition.

Rehabilitation and Physical Therapy: For elderly patients recovering from injuries or surgeries, rehabilitation and physical therapy are often necessary. Holistic care includes designing tailored rehabilitation programs to improve mobility and independence.

Medication Management: Elderly patients often take multiple medications. Holistic nursing ensures that medications are managed safely, and patients understand their medications' purposes, potential side effects, and interactions.

Advanced Care Planning: Holistic care involves discussing and documenting the elderly patient's preferences for end-of-life care, including decisions about resuscitation, life support, and hospice care if needed.

Patient and Family Education: Holistic nursing provides education to both elderly patients and their families, empowering them with knowledge about managing chronic conditions, promoting overall health, and recognizing signs of deterioration.

Palliative and End-of-Life Care: For those in the later stages of life, holistic care includes palliative care and end-of-life support. This entails managing pain and symptoms, providing emotional and spiritual support, and ensuring a dignified and comfortable transition.

Respect for Cultural and Personal Beliefs: Holistic care respects the cultural and personal beliefs of elderly patients, whether related to diet, rituals, or end-of-life preferences. These beliefs are integrated into the care plan whenever possible.

Empowerment and Autonomy: Holistic care seeks to empower elderly patients to make informed decisions about their care and maintain a sense of autonomy and control over their lives.

Holistic care for the elderly recognizes that they are individuals with unique physical, emotional, social, and spiritual needs. By addressing these needs comprehensively and compassionately, nurses can enhance the quality of life for elderly patients and promote their overall well-being.

Holistic Maternal and Newborn Care

Holistic maternal and newborn care in nursing is an approach that encompasses the physical, emotional, social, and cultural aspects of pregnancy, childbirth, and the postpartum period for both the mother and the newborn. This approach recognizes that a woman's experience during pregnancy and childbirth is not solely a medical event but also a deeply personal and transformative journey. It aims to provide comprehensive care that supports the well-being and dignity of both the mother and the newborn. Here's an overview of holistic maternal and newborn care:

Prenatal Care: Holistic care begins during pregnancy with regular prenatal check-ups. It involves monitoring the physical health of the mother, ensuring proper nutrition, and addressing any medical complications. Additionally, it considers the emotional well-being of the mother, providing support for anxiety, stress, or depression that may arise during pregnancy.

Emotional and Psychological Support: Recognizing the emotional changes and challenges that come with pregnancy and childbirth, holistic care includes emotional support and counseling. This support may extend to the partner or family members as well.

Childbirth Education: Holistic care includes childbirth education classes that prepare the mother for labor and delivery. These classes cover pain management options, birthing plans, and the emotional aspects of childbirth.

Cultural Competence: Healthcare providers practicing holistic maternal and newborn care respect the cultural and spiritual beliefs of the mother. They consider cultural traditions and customs in care decisions and respect the mother's preferences.

Birth Plan: Holistic care encourages mothers to create birth plans that outline their preferences for labor and delivery. This includes choices about pain relief, positions during labor, and other aspects of the birthing experience.

Labor Support: During labor and delivery, holistic care may involve the presence of a doula or a supportive birthing partner. These individuals provide emotional and physical support to the mother, enhancing the birthing experience.

Pain Management: Holistic care provides a range of pain management options, including pharmacological and non-pharmacological methods. These options are discussed with the mother, and her choices are respected.

Immediate Postpartum Care: After childbirth, holistic care focuses on the immediate postpartum recovery of both the mother and the newborn. This includes monitoring for any complications, providing breastfeeding support, and addressing any emotional challenges.

Breastfeeding Support: Holistic care promotes and supports breastfeeding, recognizing its benefits for both the mother and the newborn. Lactation consultants may be available to assist with breastfeeding challenges.

Newborn Care: The holistic approach extends to the care of the newborn, considering their physical, emotional, and developmental needs. Newborn screenings and assessments are conducted, and parents are educated about newborn care.

Family-Centered Care: Holistic maternal and newborn care recognizes the importance of the family in the birthing experience. It involves the partner or other family members in decision-making and care planning.

Postpartum Emotional Support: Postpartum emotional support is a vital component of holistic care. It includes monitoring for postpartum depression and providing support and resources for mothers who may experience emotional challenges.

Continuity of Care: Holistic care strives for continuity of care throughout the prenatal, birthing, and postpartum periods. This ensures that the mother and newborn receive consistent and comprehensive care.

Patient-Centered Care: Ultimately, holistic care is patient-centered, with the mother actively involved in decision-making about her care and the care of her newborn.

Holistic maternal and newborn care recognizes that pregnancy and childbirth are significant life events that encompass physical, emotional, cultural, and spiritual dimensions. This approach ensures that the care provided is respectful, supportive, and tailored to the unique needs and preferences of the mother and her newborn.

Addressing Holistic Needs of Patients with Chronic Illnesses

Nurses play a crucial role in addressing the holistic needs of patients with chronic illnesses. Chronic illnesses often have a profound impact on various aspects of a person's life, including physical health, emotional well-being, social relationships, and overall quality of life. Nurses provide comprehensive care that takes into account all these dimensions to support patients in managing their chronic conditions effectively. Here's how nurses address the holistic needs of patients with chronic illnesses:

When caring for patients with chronic illnesses, nurses consider not only the physical aspects of the illness but also the emotional, social, and spiritual dimensions of the patient's life. They start by conducting thorough assessments to gain a comprehensive understanding of the patient's condition and its impact on their life.

Education is a key component of this care. Nurses provide patients with information about their condition, available treatment options, and strategies for self-management. They empower patients to take an active role in their care and make informed decisions.

Medication management is another critical aspect. Nurses ensure that patients understand their medications, including dosages, potential side effects, and drug interactions. They stress the importance of adhering to prescribed medication regimens.

Symptom management is addressed through various strategies. Nurses help patients manage symptoms such as pain, fatigue, and discomfort, providing guidance on how to alleviate these symptoms effectively.

Chronic illnesses often come with emotional challenges like anxiety, depression, and stress. Nurses offer emotional support, sometimes referring patients for counseling or therapy to address these emotional aspects and teach coping skills.

Social support is encouraged, as chronic conditions can affect a patient's social life and relationships. Nurses advocate for patients to engage with support groups, maintain connections with loved ones, and participate in social activities that promote well-being.

Nutrition and dietary choices are also discussed, with nurses providing guidance on dietary modifications that can improve the patient's health. They help patients create meal plans that align with their condition.

Physical activity is encouraged, tailored to the patient's condition and abilities. Nurses assist patients in setting realistic exercise goals and explain the benefits of staying physically active.

Holistic pain management strategies are employed, combining medical interventions with relaxation techniques and lifestyle adjustments to alleviate chronic pain.

Spiritual needs are respected, and nurses provide spiritual support or resources as requested by the patient. Cultural sensitivity is also crucial, taking into account dietary restrictions, rituals, and cultural preferences.

Individualized self-management plans are developed in collaboration with the patient. These plans encompass medication adherence, symptom monitoring, and lifestyle modifications tailored to the patient's unique needs.

Goal setting is part of the process, with nurses working alongside patients to establish achievable goals for managing their chronic condition, improving overall well-being, and enhancing their quality of life.

Regular monitoring and follow-up are essential to track the patient's condition, assess progress, and make necessary adjustments to the care plan.

Advocacy is another role of nurses, as they stand up for patients' needs within the healthcare system, helping them access appropriate resources, treatments, and support services.

Collaboration with other healthcare professionals, such as physicians, social workers, and dietitians, ensures that care is well-coordinated and comprehensive.

Addressing the holistic needs of patients with chronic illnesses involves a comprehensive approach that takes into account the physical, emotional, social, and spiritual aspects of their condition. Nurses play a pivotal role in providing this type of care, ultimately contributing to improved health outcomes and a higher quality of life for individuals living with chronic illnesses.

Holistic Mental Health Care for Adolescents

Holistic mental health care for adolescents in nursing is an all-encompassing approach that acknowledges the interconnected nature of mental health and well-being during the adolescent years. It takes into account not only the clinical aspects of mental health but also the emotional, social, and developmental needs of adolescents. Here's an explanation of how nurses provide holistic mental health care for adolescents:

Nurses begin by recognizing that adolescence is a period of significant growth and change, both physically and emotionally. They approach adolescent mental health care with empathy and sensitivity to the unique challenges and stressors that adolescents may face.

Assessment is a fundamental step in providing holistic care. Nurses conduct comprehensive assessments to understand the adolescent's mental health status, including any signs of anxiety, depression, or other mental health conditions. They also assess the social and familial context, as family dynamics and social support play crucial roles in an adolescent's mental well-being.

Effective communication is essential. Nurses create a safe and nonjudgmental environment where adolescents feel comfortable sharing their thoughts and feelings. Open dialogue allows nurses to gain insight into the adolescent's emotional state, concerns, and stressors.

Education is a key component of holistic care. Nurses provide adolescents with information about mental health, explaining the signs and symptoms of common conditions and the importance of seeking help when needed. They also educate adolescents about healthy coping strategies and the benefits of self-care.

Collaboration is central to holistic mental health care. Nurses work closely with other healthcare professionals, such as psychologists, psychiatrists, and social workers, to develop a comprehensive care plan tailored to the adolescent's specific needs. This collaboration ensures that the adolescent receives the most appropriate and effective interventions.

Support for families is a crucial aspect of holistic care. Adolescents' mental health often impacts their families, and nurses provide guidance and resources to help families understand and support their adolescent's mental well-being.

Emotional support is offered to adolescents throughout their mental health journey. Nurses provide a listening ear, validate their feelings, and offer emotional support as they navigate their challenges. This support can be especially vital during times of crisis or when adolescents are experiencing emotional distress.

Promotion of coping skills and resilience is a key goal. Nurses help adolescents develop healthy coping strategies to manage stress, anxiety, and other emotional challenges. This may involve teaching relaxation techniques, problem-solving skills, and mindfulness practices.

Prevention and early intervention are emphasized. Nurses work to identify mental health concerns early on and implement interventions to prevent the escalation of problems. This proactive approach can help mitigate the impact of mental health issues on adolescents' lives.

Advocacy is part of the nurse's role. They advocate for adolescents' mental health needs within the healthcare system, schools, and communities. This may involve ensuring access to appropriate mental health services and challenging stigmatizing attitudes or barriers to care.

Ultimately, holistic mental health care for adolescents in nursing recognizes that mental health is influenced by a complex interplay of factors, including emotional, social, and developmental aspects. By addressing these dimensions comprehensively and compassionately, nurses can support adolescents in achieving and maintaining mental well-being during this crucial stage of life.

Chapter 7:
Cultural Competence and Diversity in Holistic Care

Understanding Cultural Differences

Understanding cultural differences in healthcare is a vital aspect of providing quality and patient-centered care. It involves recognizing and respecting the diversity of cultural backgrounds, beliefs, values, and practices that patients bring to their healthcare experiences. This understanding goes beyond mere tolerance; it is about embracing the richness of cultural diversity and tailoring care to meet the unique needs of each individual. It also involves self-awareness, openness, and a commitment to providing equitable and respectful healthcare for all, regardless of their cultural background.

Nurses who understand cultural differences:

Promote Inclusivity: They create healthcare environments that are inclusive and welcoming to individuals from various cultural backgrounds.

Recognize Biases: They are aware of their own cultural biases and actively work to mitigate any biases that may affect their interactions with patients.

Cultural Competence: They continuously educate themselves about the cultural norms, traditions, and customs related to health and illness within different cultural groups.

Tailored Care: They understand that one-size-fits-all approaches to healthcare may not be suitable for patients from diverse backgrounds and tailor care plans accordingly.

Informed Consent: They ensure that patients fully comprehend their healthcare options and provide informed consent in a way that respects cultural norms.

Cultural Humility: They approach care with cultural humility, acknowledging that they may not know everything about a patient's culture and remaining open to learning from their patients.

Ethical Considerations: They navigate ethical considerations, such as those related to cultural practices, in a manner that respects both cultural norms and ethical standards of care.

Advocacy: They advocate for patients to ensure that their cultural rights are upheld within the healthcare system and work towards equitable access to care for all patients, regardless of their cultural background.

Overall, understanding cultural differences is about fostering a healthcare environment where diversity is celebrated, cultural competence is the norm, and patients receive care that respects their individuality and cultural identities. It is a commitment to providing respectful, equitable, and patient-centered care that honors the unique perspectives and backgrounds of each patient.

Providing Culturally Sensitive Care

Providing culturally sensitive care in healthcare means offering healthcare services and treatments that are respectful, considerate, and responsive to the cultural beliefs, values, and preferences of each individual patient. This approach recognizes that culture plays a significant role in shaping a person's health perceptions, healthcare decisions, and overall well-being.

Culturally sensitive care begins with acknowledging the cultural diversity of patients and appreciating the richness it brings to the healthcare setting. It involves being aware of one's own cultural biases and stereotypes, ensuring that they do not negatively impact patient care.

Effective communication is at the heart of culturally sensitive care. Healthcare providers strive to communicate clearly and in a manner that patients can understand, taking into account language differences and the potential need for interpreters. They avoid using complex medical jargon and actively listen to patients to understand their unique concerns.

Culturally sensitive care involves tailoring healthcare plans to align with patients' cultural backgrounds. This may mean adjusting treatment plans, dietary recommendations, or care routines to accommodate cultural preferences and practices.

Obtaining informed consent is a crucial part of the process. Healthcare providers ensure that patients fully understand their treatment options, potential risks, and benefits, and that they make decisions freely and based on their cultural values.

Cultural competence is an ongoing goal. Healthcare providers continuously educate themselves about the cultural norms, traditions, and customs of different cultural groups. They strive to be knowledgeable and respectful of these diverse cultural perspectives.

Ethical considerations related to cultural practices are approached with sensitivity and respect. Healthcare providers uphold ethical standards while recognizing and honoring cultural values.

Patient-centered care is a key principle. Culturally sensitive care prioritizes the patient's values, beliefs, and preferences in decision-making. It respects the patient's cultural context and ensures that healthcare decisions are aligned with it.

Cultural humility is an essential attitude. Healthcare providers remain open to learning from their patients and their unique cultural backgrounds. They approach each patient with humility, recognizing that they may not have all the answers.

Promoting trust is fundamental to culturally sensitive care. Healthcare providers build trust with patients by demonstrating respect, empathy, and cultural competence. Patients are more likely to engage in their care when they feel understood and respected.

Advocacy may be part of the healthcare provider's role. They advocate for patients to ensure that their cultural rights are upheld within the healthcare system and work towards equitable access to care for all patients, regardless of their cultural background.

Ultimately, providing culturally sensitive care is about creating an inclusive healthcare environment where diversity is celebrated, communication is effective, and each patient receives care that respects their individuality and cultural identity. It leads to improved patient experiences, better health outcomes, and greater patient satisfaction.

The Role of Cultural Beliefs in Health

The role of cultural beliefs in health is significant and multifaceted. Cultural beliefs, often deeply rooted in traditions, values, and collective experiences, shape individuals' perceptions of health, illness, and healthcare practices. They influence how people understand, approach, and manage their health, as well as their interactions with the healthcare system. Here are some key aspects of the role of cultural beliefs in health:

Health Perceptions: Cultural beliefs strongly influence how individuals perceive health and well-being. Different cultures may have varying definitions of what constitutes good health. For example, some cultures may prioritize physical health, while others emphasize emotional or spiritual well-being.

Illness Explanations: Cultural beliefs often provide explanations for the causes of illness. These explanations can range from biomedical factors (such as infections) to cultural or supernatural causes (such as curses or imbalances in energy). Understanding these explanations is essential for healthcare providers when diagnosing and treating patients.

Health Practices: Cultural beliefs guide health-related practices, including dietary choices, exercise routines, and hygiene rituals. These practices can vary significantly between cultures and can impact overall health and well-being.

Traditional Medicine: Many cultures have their own traditional healing systems, such as traditional Chinese medicine, Ayurveda, or herbal remedies. Cultural beliefs play a central role in these practices, which are often passed down through generations.

Treatment Preferences: Cultural beliefs influence individuals' preferences for healthcare treatments. Some patients may prefer traditional or alternative therapies over Western medicine, while others may seek a combination of both.

Healthcare Decision-Making: Cultural beliefs can shape how healthcare decisions are made within families and communities. In some cultures, family members or community leaders may have a significant say in medical decisions.

Stigma and Mental Health: Cultural beliefs can contribute to the stigma associated with certain health conditions, especially mental illnesses. Misconceptions about mental health may prevent individuals from seeking treatment or disclosing their struggles.

Health Disparities: Cultural beliefs can contribute to health disparities, as individuals from different cultural backgrounds may face unique barriers to accessing healthcare services or adhering to medical recommendations.

Cultural Competence: Healthcare providers need to be culturally competent, meaning they are sensitive to and knowledgeable about the cultural beliefs of their patients. This competence enables them to provide patient-centered care that respects and incorporates cultural perspectives.

In summary, cultural beliefs are integral to a person's understanding of health, illness, and healthcare practices. Recognizing and respecting these beliefs is essential for healthcare providers to deliver effective and culturally sensitive care, ultimately leading to better health outcomes and improved patient experiences.

Overcoming Language Barriers

Overcoming language barriers is a critical aspect of providing effective and patient-centered care to individuals who speak languages different from that of the healthcare provider. Language barriers can hinder communication, compromise patient safety, and impede the understanding of important medical information. Nurses play a pivotal role in ensuring that language differences do not become barriers to quality healthcare. Here's an explanation of how nurses overcome language barriers:

Use of Professional Interpreters: Nurses recognize the importance of using professional interpreters to facilitate communication. Qualified interpreters, whether in-person, over the phone, or through video conferencing, help bridge the language gap between healthcare providers and patients.

Patient-Centered Approach: Nurses approach patients with empathy and patience, understanding that language barriers may cause frustration or anxiety for both the patient and the provider. They create a supportive and welcoming environment that encourages effective communication.

Clear and Simple Language: Nurses use clear, plain language to communicate with patients. They avoid medical jargon and complex terminology, opting for simple explanations that are easier to understand, especially for patients with limited English proficiency.

Visual Aids: Nurses may utilize visual aids such as diagrams, pictures, or charts to help convey information. Visual aids can enhance understanding and provide an additional layer of communication beyond verbal language.

Gestures and Body Language: Non-verbal communication, such as gestures and body language, can convey meanings and emotions across language barriers. Nurses use gestures thoughtfully to enhance understanding while ensuring that cultural sensitivities are respected.

Active Listening: Nurses engage in active listening by giving patients ample time to express themselves. They ask open-ended questions, provide opportunities for patients to ask questions, and carefully listen to patients' responses to ensure accurate comprehension.

Repeat and Summarize: Nurses often repeat and summarize important information to ensure that patients have grasped the content correctly. This technique helps verify comprehension and allows patients to ask for clarifications.

Avoiding Assumptions: Nurses avoid making assumptions about patients' language proficiency. Instead, they directly inquire about the patient's preferred language and ensure that appropriate language assistance is provided.

Family and Friends: While using trained interpreters is ideal, nurses may involve family members or friends who are proficient in both languages to help with communication. However, this approach should be used cautiously to maintain patient confidentiality and accuracy of information.

Multilingual Resources: Hospitals and clinics often provide multilingual resources, such as translated brochures and educational materials, to support patients' understanding of their condition, treatment, and care instructions.

Documenting Interactions: Nurses ensure that all interactions involving interpretation are properly documented in the patient's medical record. This documentation helps maintain continuity of care and ensures that accurate information is shared among healthcare providers.

Cultural Sensitivity: Nurses are culturally sensitive when overcoming language barriers. They consider cultural norms, beliefs, and values while communicating and ensure that their approach is respectful and aligned with the patient's cultural background.

Continuous Learning: Nurses seek opportunities to enhance their own language skills or learn basic phrases in languages commonly spoken by their patient population. This effort demonstrates a commitment to improving patient communication.

By employing these strategies, nurses ensure that language barriers do not compromise the quality of care they provide. Effective communication is central to building trust, fostering patient engagement, and ultimately improving health outcomes for individuals who speak different languages.

Holistic Nursing in Diverse Communities

Holistic nursing in diverse communities is an approach to healthcare that recognizes and respects the unique cultural, ethnic, and socioeconomic backgrounds of individuals within a community. It involves providing comprehensive and patient-centered care that integrates cultural sensitivity and understanding into the healthcare process. Here are some key aspects of holistic nursing in diverse communities:

Cultural Competence: Holistic nurses strive to understand the diverse cultures present in their community. For example, in a neighborhood with a significant Hispanic population, a nurse might learn about traditional healing practices, dietary preferences, and family dynamics within Hispanic culture.

Language Assistance: In communities with a variety of languages spoken, nurses ensure language barriers don't hinder care. They may use interpreters or offer translated materials. For instance, in a multicultural city, a nurse might use a professional interpreter to communicate with a patient who speaks a language different from their own.

Respect for Cultural Beliefs: Holistic nurses respect and incorporate cultural beliefs into care. For instance, if a Native American patient prefers traditional herbal remedies for pain relief, a nurse would consider these preferences while developing a pain management plan.

Individualized Care Plans: Care plans are tailored to each patient's cultural context. For instance, a nurse working in a diverse community would recognize that dietary recommendations for a patient of Indian descent might differ from those for a patient of African descent, considering cultural dietary preferences and restrictions.

Health Education: Holistic nurses provide culturally sensitive health education. In a community with a high Asian population, a nurse might create educational materials that incorporate cultural symbols and concepts relevant to that community.

Cultural Safety: The healthcare environment is designed to be culturally safe, where patients can express their concerns and beliefs without fear of judgment. For example, a nurse ensures that the clinic's waiting room includes materials and images that reflect the diversity of the community.

Collaborative Care: Nurses collaborate with other healthcare professionals and community organizations to address the unique healthcare needs of the community. For example, they may work with local cultural centers to provide health promotion workshops.

Cultural Humility: Holistic nurses approach care with humility, acknowledging that they don't know everything about every culture. They remain open to learning and adapting their care practices as they encounter new cultural perspectives.

Promotion of Wellness: In diverse communities, holistic nurses emphasize wellness and preventative care. They work with community leaders to organize health fairs and screenings tailored to the specific needs and cultural beliefs of the community.

Addressing Health Disparities: Holistic nurses are proactive in addressing health disparities that may exist within the community. They advocate for equitable healthcare access and strive to eliminate disparities related to ethnicity, culture, or socioeconomic status.

End-of-Life Care: Nurses in diverse communities understand and respect cultural differences in end-of-life care and rituals. They ensure that patients and families can observe their cultural practices and traditions during this sensitive time.

Holistic nursing in diverse communities involves providing care that is culturally sensitive, respectful, and tailored to the unique backgrounds and beliefs of the community's residents. This approach aims to enhance the overall health and well-being of individuals within diverse communities while reducing healthcare disparities and ensuring equitable access to quality care.

Chapter 8:
Holistic Self-Care for Nurses

The Importance of Self-Care

The importance of self-care cannot be overstated. Nursing is a demanding and often emotionally taxing profession that requires nurses to provide compassionate care to patients while managing the physical and emotional challenges of their work. Self-care is vital for nurses to maintain their own well-being and to continue providing high-quality care to their patients. Here's why self-care is so crucial:

Physical Health: Nursing involves long hours, physically demanding tasks, and exposure to various health risks. Proper self-care, including exercise, a balanced diet, and adequate rest, helps nurses stay physically healthy and maintain the energy required to perform their duties effectively.

Emotional Resilience: Nurses often encounter emotionally challenging situations, such as patient suffering, loss, and high-stress environments. Self-care practices like mindfulness, stress management, and seeking emotional support are essential for building emotional resilience and preventing burnout.

Mental Well-Being: The demands of nursing can lead to high levels of stress and anxiety. Engaging in self-care activities, like meditation, journaling, or seeking therapy, can help nurses manage their mental health and reduce the risk of developing conditions like depression or anxiety.

Compassion Fatigue Prevention: Compassion fatigue, also known as secondary traumatic stress, is a risk for nurses who regularly witness suffering and trauma. Self-care techniques can help nurses mitigate the emotional toll of their work and maintain their capacity for empathy and compassion.

Better Patient Care: Nurses who prioritize self-care are better equipped to provide high-quality care to their patients. When nurses are physically and mentally well, they can focus on their patients' needs, make sound clinical judgments, and offer emotional support effectively.

Reduced Burnout: Nursing is known for its high rates of burnout. Burnout can lead to increased absenteeism, decreased job satisfaction, and ultimately, leaving the profession. Self-care can significantly reduce the risk of burnout and help nurses stay engaged and fulfilled in their careers.

Enhanced Job Satisfaction: Self-care practices contribute to job satisfaction. When nurses take time to care for themselves, they are more likely to feel satisfied in their roles, which can positively impact their performance and job retention.

Positive Work-Life Balance: Nursing often involves irregular hours and shift work, making it challenging to maintain work-life balance. Self-care helps nurses establish boundaries between work and personal life, allowing them to recharge and spend quality time with loved ones.

Improved Resilience in Crisis: Healthcare crises, such as the COVID-19 pandemic, can place immense pressure on nurses. Self-care practices can equip nurses with the tools they need to endure and recover from these challenging situations.

Role Modeling: Nurses who prioritize self-care set a positive example for their colleagues and future generations of nurses. They contribute to a culture of well-being within the profession.

Self-care is not a luxury for nurses; it's a necessity. It is an essential component of maintaining physical and mental health, preventing burnout, and providing high-quality patient care. Nurses who practice self-care are better equipped to navigate the demands of their profession while enjoying fulfilling and sustainable careers.

Preventing Burnout

Preventing burnout is crucial for maintaining physical and mental well-being, both in nursing and various other professions. Burnout can lead to emotional exhaustion, reduced job satisfaction, and even long-term health issues. Here are some strategies to prevent burnout:

Set Boundaries: Establish clear boundaries between work and personal life. Avoid overextending yourself by taking on too many shifts or responsibilities. Learn to say "no" when necessary to avoid burnout.

Time Management: Efficient time management can reduce stress and prevent burnout. Prioritize tasks, delegate when possible, and organize your workload to prevent feeling overwhelmed.

Seek Support: Build a support network within your workplace and outside of it. Share your challenges and feelings with colleagues, friends, or a therapist. Connecting with others who understand the demands of nursing can be immensely beneficial.

Mentorship and Peer Support: Seek mentorship from experienced nurses who can provide guidance and share their coping strategies. Peer support groups or mentorship programs within your organization can offer valuable resources for managing stress.

Regular Breaks: Take regular breaks during your shifts to recharge. Short breaks for rest, meals, and hydration can help prevent burnout during long and demanding shifts.

Mindfulness and Stress Reduction: Practice mindfulness techniques, meditation, or deep breathing exercises to manage stress. These practices can help you stay grounded and focused, even in high-pressure situations.

Professional Development: Invest in ongoing professional development and education. Expanding your skills and knowledge can increase your confidence and job satisfaction.

Recognize Signs of Burnout: Be aware of the signs of burnout, such as chronic fatigue, irritability, decreased motivation, and changes in sleep patterns. If you notice these signs, take them seriously and seek support.

Time Off: Utilize your paid time off (PTO) and vacation days to rest and recharge.

Taking regular vacations or even short breaks can significantly reduce burnout risk.

Supervision and Management Support: Engage with your supervisors or managers to discuss workload and job-related stressors. They can provide support and solutions to help manage your responsibilities.

Advocate for Workplace Improvements: Advocate for changes in your workplace that can improve nurse well-being, such as manageable nurse-to-patient ratios, safe staffing levels, and resources for stress management.

Regular Health Checkups: Schedule regular health checkups to monitor your physical and mental health. Early intervention can prevent health issues from escalating.

Reflect on Your Career Goals: Periodically reflect on your career goals and values.

Ensure that your current role aligns with your aspirations and passions.

Take Time for Yourself: Don't forget to take time for yourself outside of work. Engage in activities that recharge you and help you disconnect from work-related stressors.

Remember that preventing burnout is an ongoing process. Regularly assess your well-being, seek support when needed, and adapt your self-care strategies to suit your changing needs. By prioritizing self-care and implementing these strategies, you can reduce the risk of burnout and enjoy a more fulfilling nursing career.

Mindfulness and Meditation for Nurses

Mindfulness and meditation are valuable practices for nurses to enhance their well-being, reduce stress, and improve their ability to provide patient-centered care.

These techniques can help nurses manage the demands of their profession, stay focused, and maintain emotional resilience. Here's how mindfulness and meditation can benefit nurses:

Stress Reduction: Nursing can be highly stressful due to long shifts, high patient loads, and emotionally taxing situations. Mindfulness and meditation techniques can help nurses manage stress and prevent burnout.

Improved Focus: Mindfulness practices, such as mindful breathing or meditation, can enhance concentration and attention. This improved focus can be particularly beneficial when administering medications, documenting patient information, or performing complex procedures.

Emotional Resilience: Mindfulness cultivates emotional resilience by helping nurses acknowledge and process their emotions in a healthy way. This can reduce the risk of compassion fatigue and secondary traumatic stress, which are common in healthcare professions.

Enhanced Communication: Mindfulness can improve communication skills by promoting active listening and empathetic responses. Nurses who practice mindfulness are better equipped to understand patients' concerns and provide compassionate care.

Pain Management: Mindfulness meditation techniques can be effective in managing pain, both for patients and nurses experiencing physical discomfort due to the demands of their work.

Improved Sleep: Many nurses work irregular hours, which can disrupt sleep patterns. Mindfulness practices can help improve sleep quality and duration by reducing insomnia and promoting relaxation.

Conflict Resolution: Mindfulness can help nurses remain calm and composed in high-stress situations, facilitating effective conflict resolution and teamwork.

Enhanced Empathy: Mindfulness promotes empathy and compassion, allowing nurses to better understand the experiences and emotions of their patients. This can lead to more patient-centered care.

Practical Tips for Nurses:

Begin with short mindfulness sessions, such as 5-10 minutes of meditation, and gradually increase the duration as you become more comfortable.

Establish a regular mindfulness practice. Consistency is key to experiencing the benefits.

Incorporate mindfulness into your daily routine. For example, practice mindful breathing during breaks or before entering a patient's room.

There are numerous mindfulness and meditation apps available that offer guided sessions tailored to healthcare professionals.

Consider attending mindfulness or stress reduction courses specifically designed for healthcare providers.

Take short mindful walks during breaks to refresh your mind and reduce stress.

Regularly reflect on the impact of mindfulness on your well-being and work performance.

Connect with colleagues who are interested in mindfulness to provide mutual support and encouragement.

By incorporating mindfulness and meditation into their lives, nurses can enhance their personal well-being, reduce stress, and become more effective and compassionate healthcare providers.

Holistic Nutrition and Exercise for Nurses

Holistic nutrition and exercise are essential components of self-care for nurses, promoting physical and mental well-being. These practices can help nurses maintain their health, boost energy levels, and better cope with the physical and emotional demands of their profession. Here's how holistic nutrition and exercise benefit nurses:

Holistic Nutrition for Nurses

Sustained Energy: Proper nutrition ensures a steady supply of energy throughout long shifts, reducing fatigue and helping nurses stay alert and focused.

Immune System Support: A well-balanced diet provides essential nutrients that support a robust immune system. This is especially important for nurses who may be exposed to various illnesses.

Mental Clarity: Nutrient-dense foods, including fruits, vegetables, and whole grains, can enhance cognitive function, improving decision-making and problem-solving abilities.

Stress Management: Certain foods, like those rich in omega-3 fatty acids (e.g., fatty fish, flaxseeds), can help reduce stress and anxiety levels.

Weight Management: Maintaining a healthy weight is essential for overall well-being. Proper nutrition can help nurses manage their weight and reduce the risk of obesity-related health issues.

Digestive Health: A diet high in fiber supports digestive health and helps prevent gastrointestinal problems, which can be exacerbated by stress.

Practical Tips for Holistic Nutrition:

- Prioritize whole, unprocessed foods, such as fruits, vegetables, lean proteins, whole grains, and legumes.
- Stay hydrated by drinking plenty of water throughout your shift.
- Plan and pack nutritious meals and snacks to avoid reliance on fast food or vending machines.
- Be mindful of portion sizes to maintain a healthy weight.
- Limit the consumption of sugary and high-caffeine beverages, as they can lead to energy crashes.

Exercise for Nurses

Physical Fitness: Regular exercise helps nurses build and maintain physical fitness, making it easier to perform physically demanding tasks and reducing the risk of injuries.

Stress Reduction: Physical activity is an excellent stress reliever, promoting the release of endorphins, which are natural mood lifters.

Improved Cardiovascular Health: Cardiovascular exercise, such as jogging or swimming, strengthens the heart and improves circulation, reducing the risk of heart disease.

Muscular Strength: Strength training exercises can enhance muscular strength, making it easier to lift and transfer patients safely.

Flexibility and Mobility: Stretching and flexibility exercises can improve range of motion and reduce the risk of musculoskeletal injuries.

Better Sleep: Regular exercise can promote better sleep quality and help nurses cope with irregular shift work.

Mental Health: Exercise is associated with reduced symptoms of depression and anxiety, providing valuable emotional support.

Practical Tips for Exercise:

- Find an exercise routine that you enjoy and can realistically incorporate into your schedule.
- Aim for at least 150 minutes of moderate-intensity aerobic exercise or 75 minutes of vigorous-intensity exercise per week.
- Incorporate strength training exercises at least two days a week.
- Take advantage of breaks during your shift to stretch and move around.
- Consider engaging in group fitness classes or activities with colleagues to

make exercise more enjoyable and social.

Incorporating holistic nutrition and regular exercise into your lifestyle can significantly enhance your overall well-being as a nurse. These practices not only benefit your physical health but also support your mental and emotional resilience, helping you provide the best care possible to your patients while maintaining your own health and vitality.

Chapter 9:
Ethical Considerations in Holistic Nursing

Ethical Principles in Nursing

Ethical principles in nursing serve as guiding frameworks to help nurses make ethical decisions and provide high-quality, patient-centered care. These principles are rooted in ethical theories and values and provide a foundation for ethical nursing practice. Here are the key ethical principles in nursing:

Autonomy: This is the principle of respecting a patient's right to make their own decisions about their healthcare. Nurses should provide patients with the information and support needed to make informed choices and respect those choices, even if they disagree with them.

Beneficence: It is the principle of doing good and acting in the best interests of the patient. Nurses have a duty to provide care that maximizes the benefits to the patient and minimizes harm.

Non-Maleficence: This is the principle of "do no harm." Nurses should avoid causing harm to patients and prioritize their safety and well-being.

Justice: It involves the fair distribution of healthcare resources and the equitable treatment of patients. Nurses should ensure that all patients receive equal and fair access to care, regardless of factors like race, gender, or socioeconomic status.

Veracity: This is the principle of truth-telling and honesty. Nurses should provide accurate and complete information to patients, respecting their right to know about their condition and treatment options.

Fidelity: It is also known as loyalty or faithfulness, refers to the nurse's obligation to be trustworthy and keep promises. Nurses should follow through on their commitments to patients and colleagues.

Confidentiality: Nurses must maintain patient confidentiality by safeguarding patient information and only sharing it with those who have a legitimate need to know for healthcare purposes.

Accountability: It involves taking responsibility for one's actions and decisions in nursing practice. Nurses should be accountable for their own actions and advocate for accountability in the healthcare system.

Respect: Respect for the dignity and worth of every individual is a fundamental ethical principle. Nurses should treat patients and colleagues with respect, regardless of their background, beliefs, or circumstances.

Cultural Competence: This involves recognizing and respecting the cultural beliefs, values, and practices of patients. Nurses should provide culturally sensitive care that acknowledges and incorporates cultural diversity.

Informed Consent: Nurses should ensure that patients provide informed consent before any medical intervention. This includes explaining the risks, benefits, and alternatives to treatment in a way the patient can understand.

Duty of Care: Nurses have a professional duty to provide care to the best of their abilities and within the scope of their practice. This includes advocating for patients and ensuring their safety.

These ethical principles provide a framework for ethical decision-making in nursing practice. Nurses often encounter complex ethical dilemmas, and these principles help guide them in making decisions that prioritize the well-being and rights of patients while upholding professional standards of care. Ethical considerations are an integral part of providing patient-centered care and maintaining the trust and integrity of the nursing profession.

Ethical Dilemmas in Holistic Care

Ethical dilemmas can arise in holistic care, just as they can in other areas of healthcare. Holistic care emphasizes the physical, mental, emotional, and spiritual aspects of a patient's well-being and often involves a more personalized and patient-centered approach. Here are some common ethical dilemmas that nurses and healthcare providers may encounter in holistic care:

Patient Autonomy vs. Beneficence: Balancing a patient's autonomy and their best interests can be challenging. For example, if a patient with a life-threatening condition refuses a particular treatment based on personal spiritual beliefs, healthcare providers may face a dilemma regarding whether to respect the patient's autonomy or prioritize beneficence by providing life-saving treatment.

Informed Consent and Cultural Beliefs: When a patient's cultural or spiritual beliefs significantly impact their treatment decisions, healthcare providers must navigate informed consent carefully. Ensuring the patient understands their options and the potential consequences while respecting their cultural beliefs can be ethically complex.

Conflict of Beliefs: Holistic care often incorporates complementary and alternative therapies. Healthcare providers may encounter ethical dilemmas when they personally disagree with or question the effectiveness of these therapies, but the patient expresses a strong preference for them.

Resource Allocation: In holistic care, patients may request therapies or interventions that are not typically covered by insurance or may be costly. Healthcare providers may face ethical dilemmas related to resource allocation and ensuring equitable access to care for all patients.

Maintaining Privacy and Confidentiality: Holistic care often involves addressing sensitive issues, such as mental health or sexual health. Healthcare providers may face ethical dilemmas in balancing the patient's need for holistic care with the duty to maintain privacy and confidentiality.

Scope of Practice: Healthcare providers must stay within their scope of practice when delivering holistic care. Ethical dilemmas may arise when a provider is asked to deliver care or therapies beyond their training and expertise, potentially endangering the patient.

Patient Education and Informed Decision-Making: Providing comprehensive education about holistic therapies and their potential benefits and risks can be challenging. Healthcare providers must ensure patients have accurate information to make informed decisions while avoiding undue influence or coercion.

Addressing ethical dilemmas in holistic care requires open communication, respect for patient autonomy, cultural competence, and a commitment to balancing the principles of beneficence and non-maleficence. Collaboration with interdisciplinary teams, ethical consultations, and ethical frameworks can also be valuable in navigating complex ethical situations in holistic care.

Chapter 10:
Holistic Nursing in the Future

The Evolution of Holistic Nursing

The evolution of holistic nursing reflects a shift in healthcare from a narrow focus on physical symptoms to a more comprehensive approach that addresses the physical, emotional, mental, and spiritual well-being of patients.

The foundations of holistic nursing can be traced back to early nursing pioneers like Florence Nightingale, who emphasized the importance of providing holistic care that considers the patient's physical, emotional, and psychological needs. Nightingale's writings and practices laid the groundwork for a more comprehensive approach to nursing care.

The modern holistic nursing movement emerged in the mid-20th century, with nurse leaders such as Martha Rogers and Margaret Newman advocating for a more holistic view of nursing. They emphasized the interconnectedness of all aspects of a person's being and the need to consider the whole person in healthcare.

In 1981, the American Holistic Nurses Association (AHNA) was founded to promote holistic nursing practice and provide resources and support for nurses interested in this approach. The AHNA has played a significant role in advancing holistic nursing.

Holistic nursing began to incorporate complementary and alternative therapies into patient care. Nurses explored practices such as acupuncture, massage therapy, aromatherapy, and herbal medicine as part of a holistic approach to healing.

Over time, holistic nursing gained recognition as a legitimate and valuable approach within mainstream healthcare. Holistic nurses have been integrated into hospitals, clinics, and community settings, working alongside conventional medical practitioners to provide patient-centered care.

Educational programs and certification in holistic nursing have become more widely available. Many nurses pursue certification through organizations like the AHNA to demonstrate their expertise in holistic nursing practice.

The field of holistic nursing has grown in terms of research and evidence-based practice. Studies have explored the effectiveness of holistic interventions in managing pain, reducing stress, improving patient outcomes, and enhancing overall well-being.

Holistic nursing places a strong emphasis on patient-centered care, involving patients in their care plans, respecting their autonomy, and considering their unique physical, emotional, mental, and spiritual needs.

Holistic nursing principles have been incorporated into various nursing specialties, such as psychiatric-mental health nursing, pediatric nursing, and hospice and palliative care. These specialties recognize the importance of addressing the holistic needs of patients.

Holistic nursing embraces cultural competence, recognizing the diversity of patients and respecting their cultural, spiritual, and belief systems.

The importance of holistic self-care for nurses has gained prominence. Nurses are encouraged to care for their own physical, emotional, and spiritual well-being to prevent burnout and provide better care to their patients.

The evolution of holistic nursing reflects a broader understanding of healthcare that considers the whole person and recognizes the interconnectedness of physical, emotional, mental, and spiritual well-being. Holistic nursing has become an integral part of modern healthcare, promoting healing, well-being, and quality of life for patients.

Innovations in Holistic Care

Innovations in holistic care reflect a growing recognition of the importance of addressing the physical, emotional, mental, and spiritual well-being of individuals in healthcare. These innovations have emerged in response to evolving patient needs and an increasing emphasis on patient-centered care. Here are some key innovations in holistic care:

Integrative Medicine Centers: Integrative medicine combines conventional medical treatments with complementary and alternative therapies. Integrative medicine centers have emerged, offering services such as acupuncture, massage therapy, yoga, and nutrition counseling alongside conventional medical treatments. These centers provide patients with a more holistic approach to healing.

Mindfulness and Meditation Programs: Mindfulness-based interventions and meditation programs are increasingly integrated into healthcare settings. These practices help patients manage stress, reduce anxiety, and improve overall well-being. Healthcare providers may recommend mindfulness and meditation as part of holistic care plans.

Holistic Nursing Certification: Many nurses pursue certification in holistic nursing through organizations like the American Holistic Nurses Association (AHNA). Holistic nursing certification programs provide nurses with specialized training in holistic care principles and practices, enhancing their ability to provide comprehensive care.

Whole-Person Assessment Tools: Healthcare providers are using comprehensive assessment tools that consider the physical, emotional, mental, and spiritual dimensions of a patient's health. These tools help identify areas of concern and guide personalized care plans that address the whole person.

Cultural Competence Training: Cultural competence has become a central focus in healthcare. Training programs help healthcare providers understand and respect the diverse cultural, spiritual, and belief systems of patients. This ensures that care is tailored to individual needs and preferences.

Patient-Centered Medical Homes: The patient-centered medical home model emphasizes coordinated, holistic care. In these models, healthcare teams work collaboratively to address all aspects of a patient's health, providing comprehensive support and care management.

Telehealth and Remote Monitoring: Telehealth technologies and remote monitoring tools enable patients to access holistic care from the comfort of their homes. Patients can receive virtual consultations, access wellness resources, and receive ongoing support for their physical and emotional well-being.

Holistic Cancer Care Centers: Cancer treatment centers increasingly offer holistic care services to support patients through their cancer journey. These services may include counseling, nutritional support, pain management, and complementary therapies to enhance overall well-being.

Spiritual Care Integration: Spiritual care is being integrated into healthcare settings, with chaplains and spiritual counselors providing support to patients and families. This recognizes the importance of addressing patients' spiritual needs as part of holistic care.

Education and Training Programs: Holistic care education and training programs for healthcare providers are expanding. These programs teach providers about holistic principles, patient-centered care, and the integration of complementary therapies.

Patient Education and Self-Care: Holistic care emphasizes patient education and self-care. Patients are encouraged to take an active role in their well-being, with healthcare providers providing resources and guidance for self-care practices.

Research and Evidence-Based Practice: Research in the field of holistic care continues to grow, providing a stronger evidence base for holistic interventions. Evidence-based practices help ensure that holistic care approaches are effective and safe.

Innovations in holistic care are advancing the field, enhancing the quality of care, and promoting the overall well-being of patients. These innovations recognize that addressing the physical, emotional, mental, and spiritual aspects of health is essential for providing comprehensive and patient-centered care.

Integrating Technology into Holistic Nursing

Integrating technology into holistic nursing can enhance patient care, streamline processes, and improve communication among healthcare providers. While holistic nursing traditionally emphasizes the whole person, incorporating technology can complement this approach by providing tools for better assessment, communication, education, and patient engagement. Here are ways technology can be integrated into holistic nursing:

Electronic Health Records (EHRs): EHR systems allow holistic nurses to access comprehensive patient information, including physical health, mental health, and social history, in one place. This holistic view enables more personalized care planning.

Telehealth and Virtual Consultations: Telehealth platforms enable holistic nurses to conduct virtual consultations with patients, addressing their physical, emotional, and mental health needs remotely. This can improve access to care, especially for patients in remote areas.

Mobile Health (mHealth) Apps: Holistic nurses can recommend mHealth apps to patients for tracking their physical health (e.g., fitness, nutrition), mental health (e.g., mood tracking, meditation), and overall well-being. These apps can encourage self-care and provide valuable data for assessment.

Patient Portals: Patient portals allow patients to access their medical records, review test results, and communicate with healthcare providers. Holistic nurses can use portals to share educational materials and resources to support the patient's holistic well-being.

Wearable Devices: Wearable devices like fitness trackers and smartwatches can monitor physical health parameters (e.g., heart rate, activity levels), providing real-time data that holistic nurses can use for assessment and patient education.

Remote Monitoring: For patients with chronic conditions or those recovering from surgery, remote monitoring devices can transmit vital signs and health data to healthcare providers, enabling timely interventions and holistic care management.

Online Holistic Health Education: Holistic nurses can leverage online platforms and educational resources to provide patients with information on holistic wellness practices, including nutrition, stress management, and mindfulness.

Electronic Medication Reminders: Technology-based medication reminders can help patients adhere to their treatment plans, whether for physical or mental health conditions, supporting their holistic care.

Social Media and Support Groups: Online communities and social media platforms can serve as spaces for patients to connect with others who share similar health concerns, fostering emotional and mental well-being.

Videoconferencing for Group Therapy: Holistic nurses can conduct group therapy or support sessions via videoconferencing platforms, allowing patients to engage in emotional and mental health support in a virtual setting.

Telepsychiatry and Telecounseling: Telepsychiatry and telecounseling services enable holistic nurses to connect patients with mental health professionals, making emotional and mental health support more accessible.

Artificial Intelligence (AI) and Predictive Analytics: AI algorithms can analyze patient data to identify trends or potential health issues, helping holistic nurses provide proactive care. Predictive analytics can also assist in identifying patients at risk for specific health concerns.

While integrating technology into holistic nursing can offer numerous benefits, it's crucial to maintain a patient-centered approach. Holistic nurses should ensure that technology enhances, rather than replaces, the human connection and holistic care principles that underpin their practice. Additionally, respecting patient privacy and security when using technology is essential to maintain trust and confidentiality.

Emerging Trends in Mind-Body-Spirit Healthcare

Emerging trends in mind-body-spirit healthcare reflect a growing recognition of the interconnectedness of physical, mental, emotional, and spiritual well-being in healthcare practices. These trends prioritize holistic care and patient-centered approaches. Here are some notable emerging trends in mind-body-spirit healthcare:

Integrative Medicine Centers: Integrative medicine combines conventional medical treatments with complementary and alternative therapies. Integrative medicine centers are increasingly popular, offering services such as acupuncture, chiropractic care, mindfulness, yoga, and nutrition counseling alongside traditional medical treatments.

Mindfulness-Based Interventions: Mindfulness practices, such as meditation, mindfulness-based stress reduction (MBSR), and mindfulness-based cognitive therapy (MBCT), are gaining recognition in healthcare. These interventions help patients manage stress, anxiety, depression, and pain while promoting overall well-being.

Art and Music Therapy: Art and music therapy are being integrated into healthcare settings to support emotional and mental health. These creative therapies offer patients a non-verbal outlet for expression and healing.

Ecotherapy and Nature-Based Healing: Ecotherapy, also known as nature therapy, involves outdoor activities and immersion in nature to improve mental health and well-being. It recognizes the healing power of the natural world and is being incorporated into mental health treatments.

Energy Medicine: Energy-based therapies, such as Reiki and therapeutic touch, are gaining popularity as complementary approaches to promote healing by balancing the body's energy systems.

Spiritual Care Integration: Healthcare settings increasingly recognize the importance of addressing patients' spiritual and existential needs. Chaplains, spiritual counselors, and interfaith teams are providing spiritual support alongside medical care.

Virtual Reality (VR) Therapy: VR therapy is being used for pain management, anxiety reduction, and relaxation. Patients can experience immersive environments designed to promote mental and emotional well-being.

Holistic Mental Health Programs: Holistic mental health programs consider the whole person and focus on the integration of physical, emotional, mental, and spiritual well-being in the treatment of mental health disorders.

Narrative Medicine: Narrative medicine emphasizes the importance of patients sharing their stories, which can help healthcare providers better understand patients' experiences and support their mental and emotional health.

Psychedelic-Assisted Therapy: Research into the therapeutic use of psychedelics, such as psilocybin and MDMA, for conditions like PTSD and depression is growing. These substances are being studied for their potential to facilitate transformative and spiritually significant experiences.

Telehealth and Digital Well-Being: Telehealth platforms and digital wellness apps offer mental health and wellness support, making care more accessible and convenient.

Cultural Competence and Diversity: Healthcare providers are placing greater emphasis on cultural competence and recognizing the diverse spiritual and cultural backgrounds of patients to provide more personalized care.

Whole-Person Assessment Tools: Advanced assessment tools consider not only physical health but also emotional, mental, and spiritual well-being. These tools help healthcare providers develop comprehensive care plans.

Peer Support and Community-Based Care: Peer support programs and community-based initiatives provide patients with connections to others who have similar health concerns, offering emotional and mental support.

These emerging trends reflect a shift toward a more holistic approach in healthcare that recognizes the importance of addressing the mind, body, and spirit to promote overall well-being and healing. As these trends continue to evolve, they are likely to play a significant role in shaping the future of healthcare practices and patient-centered care.

The Ongoing Importance of Holistic Nursing Care

Holistic nursing care continues to be of paramount importance in modern healthcare for several compelling reasons:

Holistic nursing emphasizes the whole person, addressing not only physical symptoms but also emotional, mental, and spiritual needs. This comprehensive approach ensures that patients receive care tailored to their unique circumstances, resulting in better outcomes and improved patient satisfaction.

By addressing the mind, body, and spirit, holistic nursing promotes overall well-being and supports the body's natural healing processes. Patients often experience improved physical and mental health, reduced stress, and a higher quality of life.

Holistic care encourages active participation and collaboration between healthcare providers and patients. Patients who feel heard and respected in their holistic care are more likely to engage in their treatment plans and adhere to recommendations.

Holistic nursing incorporates preventive care strategies that focus on maintaining health and preventing illness. By addressing lifestyle factors, nutrition, and stress management, holistic care can help prevent chronic diseases and promote long-term health.

The growing awareness of the impact of mental health on physical health underscores the importance of addressing emotional and mental well-being in healthcare. Holistic nursing recognizes this connection and provides support for mental health concerns.

Holistic nursing takes into account each patient's unique values, beliefs, and preferences. This personalized approach ensures that care plans align with the patient's goals and values, fostering trust and cooperation.

In an increasingly diverse world, cultural competence is vital in healthcare. Holistic nursing acknowledges the diverse cultural backgrounds of patients and seeks to provide culturally sensitive care that respects individual beliefs and practices.

Holistic approaches to pain management, such as mindfulness and complementary therapies, offer alternatives to traditional pain management techniques. These approaches can reduce the reliance on opioids and minimize the risk of addiction.

Holistic nursing helps patients develop resilience and coping skills to navigate life's challenges, reducing the negative impact of stress and adversity on health.

Holistic self-care is equally important for healthcare providers. Holistic nursing encourages nurses and other healthcare professionals to prioritize their well-being, preventing burnout and ensuring they can provide compassionate care to patients.

Patients who receive holistic care often report higher levels of satisfaction and trust in their healthcare providers. This positive relationship can lead to improved patient outcomes and better healthcare experiences.

Holistic nursing continues to evolve with advances in research and healthcare innovation. New evidence-based practices and therapies are being developed to enhance holistic care and its effectiveness.

Holistic nursing care remains crucial in modern healthcare due to its patient-centered approach, emphasis on overall well-being, and ability to address the complex interplay of physical, emotional, mental, and spiritual factors in health and healing. As healthcare evolves, the ongoing importance of holistic nursing care is likely to become even more pronounced, contributing to improved patient outcomes and a more compassionate healthcare system.

Conclusion

Holistic nursing care, which integrates the dimensions of mind, body, and spirit, stands as a beacon of patient-centered healthcare in our increasingly complex and interconnected world. It recognizes that individuals are not just physical bodies with ailments but complex beings with unique emotional, mental, and spiritual needs. This holistic approach emphasizes the interconnectedness of these aspects and their profound influence on health and healing.

Holistic nursing care empowers healthcare providers to go beyond the diagnosis and treatment of diseases, allowing them to engage in a deeper, more meaningful relationship with their patients. It fosters a sense of trust, respect, and collaboration, where patients actively participate in their care decisions, and their values and beliefs are honored.

In a healthcare landscape that often focuses on symptom management and quick fixes, holistic nursing care serves as a reminder of the enduring importance of patient well-being and quality of life. It recognizes that healing extends beyond the alleviation of physical pain to encompass emotional and spiritual comfort.

As healthcare continues to evolve, the principles of holistic nursing care remain not only relevant but increasingly vital. They contribute to a more compassionate and patient-centered healthcare system, where individuals are treated with dignity and where the journey to health is characterized by understanding, empathy, and a commitment to addressing the entirety of human existence — mind, body, and spirit. In essence, holistic nursing care illuminates the path towards a more holistic, humane, and effective approach to healthcare.

- THE END -

www.ingramcontent.com/pod-product-compliance
Lightning Source LLC
Chambersburg PA
CBHW072149290526
45794CB00004B/1457